At some point there has to be peace and quiet!

Peter Caspari • Helga Dill
Cornelia Caspari • Gerhard
Hackenschmied

At some point there has to be peace and quiet!

Institutional struggle to working through the past of sexual violence and abuse of power at an institute for analytical child and adolescent psychotherapy

Springer

Peter Caspari
Institute of Practice Research and Project Consulting (IPP)
Munich, Germany

Helga Dill
Institute of Practice Research and Project Consulting (IPP)
Munich, Germany

Cornelia Caspari
Psychological Psychotherapist
Munich, Germany

Gerhard Hackenschmied
Institute of Practice Research and Project Consulting (IPP)
Munich, Germany

ISBN 978-3-658-39784-5 ISBN 978-3-658-39785-2 (eBook)
https://doi.org/10.1007/978-3-658-39785-2

This Springer imprint is published by the registered company Springer Fachmedien Wiesbaden GmbH, part of Springer Nature.
The registered company address is: Abraham-Lincoln-Str. 46, 65189 Wiesbaden, Germany

Foreword

How do social developments arise? How can one explain that there are always changes in social consciousness, that suddenly abusive relationships can be seen and named, over which a cloak of silence had previously been spread for decades? In the 1960s, the paediatrician Henry Kempe (Kempe et al., 1962) "discovered" a "new" clinical picture in the USA: The battered child syndrome, i.e. the typical consequences of child abuse, which had been overlooked by paediatricians until then; after its publication, the number of reported cases increased by leaps and bounds and exponentially: Awareness of the existence of child abuse had been awakened, so to speak. For family sexual abuse, there was such a change of consciousness in Europe in the mid-1980s (cf. Hirsch, 1987/1999); suddenly the media, the judiciary, and finally also the psychotherapeutic and psychoanalytic professionals and their organizations were able to name the true circumstances. In 1999, the Frankfurter Rundschau published a full-page article reporting on the numerous cases of sexual abuse of students of the well-known reform pedagogical Odenwald School by its director, as well as on the culture of abuse at this school. And the reaction of society? The article was not taken note of in any way, not by any media, not by local and national politics, not even by law enforcement agencies. In the same way, it was impossible to perceive and name the horrendous abuse conditions in the churches, especially in the Catholic Church, until 2010, when the Jesuit priest Klaus Mertes, due to the demands of those affected, could not help but initiate the disclosure of sexual abuse in the Canisius College in Berlin, thus giving the impetus for a broad public confrontation with the mass sexual abuse of wards in religious institutions. As a result, society could no longer close its eyes to the conditions in the well-known reform pedagogical school; the so-called Me Too movement can be understood as another area of this development.

And now some psychoanalytic training institutes are also drawing attention to themselves in the same way. These are by no means unaffected by social tendencies and developments. Even if sexuality is (was?) the genuine core of Freudian psychoanalysis, the topic of love in analysis (the title of the 1996 conference of the German Society for Psychoanalysis and Depth Psychology, DGPT) was rather disregarded. In the 1980s, there was an accumulation of international publications on this subject, in Germany the DGPT conference mentioned above, at which the psychoanalyst Günter Bittner wanted to explicitly legitimize sexual relationships between analyst and analysand or patient (cf. Hirsch, 1998), incidentally with exactly the same arguments that the protagonist of the present study used: the relationship of two adults was nobody's business. The conflict over this provocation led to a symposium of the DGPT in 1998, where the question of abstinence and the problem of sexualized abuse of power were thoroughly discussed. In this sense, the events at the AKJP Institute in Heidelberg were able to remain without consequences for many years, also due to the ignorance in society and specialist public that prevailed until the 1990s.

Psychoanalysis arose – not to be forgotten – from Freud's discovery of the pathogenic relevance of child sexual abuse in the family. (However, Freud abandoned this seduction theory in 1897 in favour of an – oedipal – drive psychology.) Freud developed his theories on the basis of his experiences with his female patients; he himself called the corresponding publications "Novellen" (Novellas), they were case stories whose reception in subsequent generations of psychoanalysts led to ever new theoretical ideas. The most impressive, harrowing news of sexualized, narcissistic abuse of power in analyses and psychotherapies has come to us through the accounts of those affected: Anonyma (1988), Joëlle Augerolles (1989/1990), Christa v. Petersdorff (2003), Margarete Akoluth (2004). The present volume, however, is not a case story, but rather the result of a socio-psychological investigation which, using scientific methods of social psychology and organizational dynamics, thoroughly examines the scandalous, decades-long abuse in a psychoanalytic training institute (for analytical child and adolescent psychotherapy) on the basis of a contemporary psychoanalytic understanding.

How could a perpetrator of abuse go on almost unnoticed for so long? Individual, group- and organizational dynamic factors came together. The perpetrator came from the outside as the saviour of an almost failed institute and was therefore already idolized and idealized, he uncontrollably united in his person a manifold formal and psychological abundance of power, he established a network of nepotism of dependents. Typical fears and resistances arose to recognize, name and expose the increasingly obvious abuse, fears that were to be overcome with the help of denial, cover-up, rationalization, trivialization and forgetting; the primary goal was to preserve the reputation and ultimately the existence of the institute. We know this from abusive families, from pedagogical and religious institutions: the whole is protected, the victim sacrificed once again. The central means for this was a "functional pragmatism", as the authors call it, which is based on an identification with the (powerful) aggressor; accordingly, empathy and identification with the victims were missing throughout, just as in the aforementioned organizations. The almost tragic pseudo-paradox is that it is precisely the denial and cover-up that can lead to the institution's demise, i.e. that what is feared is brought about by the very behaviour that should prevent it.

Typically, the exposure of the culture of abuse in institutions causes a group-dynamic split into a part that continues to idealize the perpetrator, upholds his merits and trivializes his deeds, and another part that strives to clarify and acknowledge the reality. If an integration of these divided subgroups through (of course fierce emotional) confrontation (also through external help) does not succeed, the institute cannot survive, as was the case with the Odenwald School as well as with the Munich-based psychoanalytic institute. The fact that in the present case only a few victims were willing to participate in working through the past suggests continuing loyalties and identifications, also particular fears of losing (professional) group membership. This circumstance plays a minor role for victims of power abuse in religious and educational institutions.

Nowadays, there are ethical guidelines everywhere in psychoanalytic institutes, and professional associations, ethics committees, ombudsmen, and chambers of physicians and psychotherapists have greater awareness. However, the authors of this book rightly demand that not only formal norms of behaviour and institutions to monitor them are necessary, but in the sense of real prevention a change of consciousness in psychoanalytic and other institutions, a change of organizational and group culture is also essential. In the first place, in training, it should be natural to talk about love and dependence in training relationships, as well as about power and narcissistic and sexualized abuse of power. What can be talked about does not have to be acted out.

The evolution of social consciousness has made the commission of this study possible, and the book will in turn contribute to a further shift in consciousness.

Heiligengrabe-Jabel (Brandenburg), Germany Mathias Hirsch

References

Akoluth, M. (2004). *Unordnung und spätes Leid.* Königshausen & Neumann.

Anonyma. (1988). *Verführung auf der Couch.* Kore.

Augerolles, J. (1990). *Mein Analytiker und ich. Tagebuch einer verhängnisvollen Beziehung.* Fischer (Erstveröffentlichung 1989).

Hirsch, M. (1998). Überlegungen zum Wesen der Analyse, zum analytischen Raum und zur Überschreitung seiner Grenzen. Eine Erwiderung auf „Liebe in der Analyse – ein Fall für den Staatsanwalt?" von Günther Bittner. *Forum der Psychoanalyse, 14,* 312–318.

Hirsch, M. (1999). *Realer Inzest. Psychodynamik des sexuellen Missbrauchs in der Familie* (3., überarbeitete Aufl.). Unveränd. Neuaufl. Psychosozial-Verlag (Erstveröffentlichung 1987).

Kempe, C. H., Solverman, F. N., Steele, B. F., Droegemueller, W., Silver, H. K. (1962). The battered child syndrome. *Journal of the American Medical Association, 181,* 17–24.

Petersdorff, C. V. (2003). *Anonyma: Verführung auf der Couch. Eine Niederschrift.* Psychosozial-Verlag (Erstveröffentlichung 1988).

Preliminary Note

But nothing is probably more urgent than the application of psychoanalytic insights to one's own group as well. One may be certain that an initial dishonesty through stubborn cover-up and concealment will eventually be passed on to the following generation as a distressing legacy. (Annemarie Dührssen, 1994)

This quotation by Annemarie Dührssen refers to the National Socialist past of German psychoanalysis and some of its representatives. Nevertheless, it can be extended to the handling of the transgression of boundaries – abstinence violations – that have taken place or are taking place in the context of psychotherapy.

In the following, we discuss the boundary violations, the sexual violence, which were committed in the AKJP-Heidelberg (Institut für analytische Kinder- und Jugendpsychotherapie) (Institute for Analytical Child and Adolescent Psychotherapy) in the years from 1975 to 1993 by the medical director and chairman at that time H. M.[1] and which are casting a shadow on the institute for nearly 30 years.

When the rumors became unmistakable, when victims turned to the management of the Institute for Psychoanalysis and Psychotherapy Heidelberg-Mannheim e.V. (IPP-Heidelberg-Mannheim),[2] when the former patient was pregnant for the second time by H. M. and was married, there were first attempts of disclosure and clarification. From then on, a disturbed institute tried again and again to unleash initiatives to clarify H. M.'s boundary violations. And again and again, the attempts reached deadlock. Some were able to hide behind a persistent secrecy of the

[1] Out of consideration for H. M.'s family, we do not mention his name in this report, but anonymize him as well as the names of all participants and interview partners.

[2] H. M. was also involved in various positions in the IPP-Heidelberg-Mannheim, see Sect. 1.2.

victims, others worried about the institute, so that the initiatives of enlightenment, which flared up again and again over the years, ultimately petered out and the extent of his boundary violations remained speculation.

H. M. left the AKJP-Heidelberg Institute in 1993, later also the association, but was able to continue practicing and working as an expert witness without being bothered. In 2017, H. M. was sentenced to probation for multiple sexual abuse of his granddaughter. In the context of this trial and on the occasion of an article in the *ZEIT* on the "Causa H. M.," the general meeting of the AKJP-Heidelberg association decided to have the incidents investigated externally. With this decision, the AKJP-Heidelberg took a courageous path of working through the past. Sexual violence and sexual exploitation occur again and again in psychotherapeutic settings. However, the affected institutions very rarely dare to take the step of an external inquiry, especially without pressure from the victims, which in other contexts, such as the religious institutions, first led to projects of working through the past of sexual violence.

The now available report documents for the first time all verifiable boundary violations of H. M. during his time as medical director of the AKJP-Heidelberg and is able to release them from the aggregate condition of rumor.

This work would not have been possible without the willingness of many people to provide information, especially former and current training candidates and members of the AKJP-Heidelberg and the IPP-Heidelberg-Mannheim, the victims who managed to talk about their experiences and the contemporary witnesses, and experts who answered our questions. We would like to thank them very much. We would also like to express our gratitude for the support of the AKJP-Heidelberg, who accompanied our study in the Advisory Group, supported it, and actively helped us to find interview partners. Our respect and gratitude also go to the family of H. M., especially to his widow, who provided us with important and insightful information and documents.

Sexual violence in psychotherapy is still a topic that is scarcely discussed in public discourse. It is difficult for the victims to find contact points. Often the hurdles are so high that the already vulnerable patients shy away from reporting or legal proceedings. With this report we hope not only to clear the fog in front of the history of the AKJP-Heidelberg but also give an impulse to the social discussion about the victims of sexual violence in psychotherapeutic relationships.

Munich, Germany Peter Caspari
Munich, Germany Helga Dill
Munich, Germany Cornelia Caspari
Munich, Germany Gerhard Hackenschmied
March 2021

Contents

1 The Context

1.1 The AKJP-Heidelberg

The AKJP-Heidelberg is a training institute for child and adolescent psychotherapy based on analytic and depth psychology. The institute is supported by the association "Institut für Analytische Kinder- und Jugendlichen-Psychotherapie Heidelberg e. V." (Institute for Analytical Child and Adolescent Psychotherapy Heidelberg), which was founded in 1949. The association currently has 110 members. The Institute includes a psychotherapeutic outpatient clinic and a educational counselling center at three locations in and around Heidelberg. In addition, the Institute has been involved in research projects in cooperation with the University of Heidelberg, among others, for many years. Numerous publications are available on this subject (see AKJP, n.d.).

The AKJP-Heidelberg is a successor institution of the Institute for Psychagogy founded by Annemarie Sänger after the war, a educational counselling center with depth psychological parent counselling and child psychotherapy. At that time, child psychotherapy was still practiced by psychagogues.

The (re)introduction of psychagogy in Germany began in Berlin at the then Institute of the DPG (Deutsche Psychoanalytische Gesellschaft, German Psychoanalytic Society). Harald Schultz-Hencke and Felix Böhm, among others, were instrumental in this.

Psychagogy was conceptually pragmatically oriented. "It is interesting to see that the psychoanalytic tradition of the old Berlin Institute from the 1920s was not taken up here; rather, a more practice-oriented profession oriented towards social therapy was created, the model for which was the work of the social workers at the Child Guidance Clinics in the USA and England, which are roughly comparable to

P. Caspari et al., *At some point there has to be peace and quiet!*,
https://doi.org/10.1007/978-3-658-39785-2_1

our present-day educational counselling centres" (Böhm 1952; quoted after Diepold, 1994).

Psychagogues had a basic pedagogical qualification and, building on this, completed a psychotherapeutic training with teaching analysis, theoretical specialist training and practical guidance. The training was long and demanding, yet the finished psychagogues were not allowed to treat alone. Psychagogy was rather understood as a medical assisting profession. "... the psychagogues, on the other hand, with an hourly limit of 35 h, were supposed to take care of the milder disorders, not treat them, mind you (...) Psychagogues were trained for something they were ultimately not allowed to practice." (Diepold, 1994). Moreover, in these early years, training was entirely in the hands of adult analysts. Both the theoretical training and the teaching analysis were offered exclusively by adult analysts. In Heidelberg, the Institute for Psychotherapy and Psychoanalysis Heidelberg-Mannheim (IPP-Heidelberg-Mannheim) took over this role.[1]

Barbara Diepold sees in this history of origins the roots for the fact that psychagogues had to struggle with a low social prestige, which even their successor, analytical child and youth therapy, has not overcome.

In 1975 the professional title was changed: the psychagogues became analytical child and adolescent psychotherapists (cf. Diepold, p. 7).

This development led to the Institute for Psychagogy Heidelberg changing its name to the Institute for Analytical Child and Adolescent Psychotherapy. However, the dependence on medicine still remained. From 1971, the psychotherapeutic treatment of children and adolescents was recognized as a health insurance benefit under certain conditions. This meant, however, that psychoanalytically trained physicians were necessary for the management of a training institute and for practical training.

H. M. held this position in the AKJP-Heidelberg from 1975 to 1993.

[1] The IPP-Heidelberg-Mannheim was founded in 1969 as a psychoanalytic training institute in the tradition of Erich Fromm, Frieda Fromm-Reichmann and Viktor v. Weizsäcker, among others. In the post-war period, the "Heidelberg School" emerged, which focused on the interfaces between psychosomatic medicine and psychoanalysis. Alexander Mitscherlich played a prominent role in this discourse. From the beginning, the IPP-Heidelberg-Mannheim saw itself as emancipatory, even subversive in its rejection of dogmatic concepts. Rather, it propagated a diversity of concepts and attitudes in psychoanalysis. (https://ipp-heidelberg.de/ueber-uns/selbstverstaendnis/)

1.2 Who Was H. M.?

H. M., born in Munich in 1932, studied medicine in Tubingen, Munich and Berlin and eventually became a specialist in paediatrics. In 1966 he moved from the children's clinic/child psychiatry in Kiel to Berlin. There he began psychotherapeutic training at the Institut für Psychotherapie e. V. Koserstraße (Institute for Psychotherapy) and at the same time completed the practical year in psychiatry. This was followed by a position at the AOK Institute, which was then headed by Annemarie Dührssen. In 1970 he became head of the children's department of the Institute for Psychogenic Diseases of the AOK. In 1971 he passed – together with J. S. – the exam to become a psychoanalyst.

In his unpublished memoirs, H. M. writes self-critically and probably with apologetic intent about his analytical training:

> By the time of the 1971 exam – you had to have treated 6 cases – I had treated 4 child cases and only 2 adult cases. We were not told about the problems in treating adults, for example transference love and its counterpart, countertransference love especially in men treating young women. Moreover, Mrs. Dührssen transferred her pronounced narcissism to her students as well. If one was employed by her at the institute, or if she had controlled most of the treatments, she liked to overestimate the abilities of her students and then, of course, they overestimated themselves. Although as a pediatrician I had an advantage in treating children, because I already had some command of the language of children in the various age groups, it was a disadvantage for me as a psychoanalyst that I had treated only two adults under control by the time of my exams. I later became a teaching analyst in Heidelberg in 1975 without having had sufficient experience in treating adults.

In 1975 H. M. moved to Heidelberg, where he took over the direction of the Institute for Psychagogy – as successor to Annemarie Sänger and Karl Tornow. The initiative for this change came from Prof. M. P., the full professor for child psychiatry in Heidelberg.

The institute – today the Institute for Analytical Child and Adolescent Therapy Heidelberg e. V. – consisted at that time of an educational counselling center and a training institute where teachers, social workers and social pedagogues were trained to become psychagogues in 4–5 years while simultaneously working.

As described above, psychagogy was initially more of a medical assistant profession. Until 1993, the *Delegationsverfahren* – a delegation procedure – applied, according to which a doctor had to examine the children and then delegate them to the therapists for treatment. Therefore, at that time it was absolutely necessary for the Institute to have a medical director. According to the statutes, the director was also the chairperson of the association. Thus, this position was associated with a considerable amount of power.

Furthermore, H. M. was also a member of the adult institute, the IPP-Heidelberg-Mannheim. He was a lecturer, teaching analyst and later also chairman of the training committee there.

In 1993, H. M. was dismissed from his leadership function during a general meeting of the AKJP-Heidelberg, after there had been accusations and rumours in connection with abstinence violations in the form of sexual boundary violations/sexual violence and a sexual relationship with a former patient could be proven. Due to this, H. M. had already resigned as a member of the IPP-Heidelberg-Mannheim. In 1999, H. M. terminated his membership in the AKJP-Heidelberg. Before that there were considerations to exclude him from his membership because of abstinence violations. The accusations and rumours referred to training candidates, patients as well as children and adolescents, girls and boys, who had experienced borderline violations by H. M. in the context of second sight (i.e. assessing the child in order to verify the diagnosis assigned by the training candidate) or the examinations in the context of the delegation procedure.

In 2017, H. M. was sentenced to probation for sexually abusing his granddaughter.

The case of H. M. has occupied the AKJP-Heidelberg since the 1990s again and again and in various forms. While H. M. had supporters for a long time who relativized his boundary violations and sexual violence, there were at the same time various attempts to working through them. Nevertheless, the rumors kept the upper hand, were passed down through the various generations of trainees and the facts about H. M. were not taken note of.

"Thus the case of H. M. remained like an abscess, which had encapsulated itself under the skin, was isolated there, but could break open at any time to threaten the whole organism".[2] A professional confrontation, e.g. with the help of external group supervision and a systematic inquiry (with the help of external experts) was nevertheless avoided over the decades.

[2] From a motion to the June 1998 General Membership Meeting to the members of the Board of Directors.

2 The Study

2.1 How the Commissioning Came About

In connection with the trial in 2017, the case of H. M. became virulent again for the AKJP-Heidelberg. Once again, a working group of enlightened people was formed, which sought answers to the following two guiding questions: (1) "How can the H. M. period and the attempts to overcome it be told, when the history of the institute is told? (2) How can this period be integrated into the history of the Institute?"

At the general meeting of the AKJP-Heidelberg in June 2018, it was decided to scientifically work through the "Causa H. M." or "Era H. M.". Subsequently, the then ethics officer of the institute contacted the IPP Munich.

At a meeting on 6 September 2018 with representatives of the IPP Munich and the working group "Causa H. M." as well as the board of AKJP-Heidelberg, the research question was specified. In April 2019, the IPP Munich started its work.

The focus of the study is the period from 1975 to 1993, i.e. the era of H. M. For a comprehensive working through of the subject of sexualised violence within the AKJP-Heidelberg, however, possible further indications of other cases of sexualised violence within the AKJP-Heidelberg should also be investigated.

The following questions guided the scientific analysis:

- What extent of sexualised violence by H.M. within the AKJP-Heidelberg can be proven?
- What structures within the Institute have encouraged this violence and hindered its detection?
- How is the handling of known and suspected cases of sexualised violence by the people in charge belonging to AKJP-Heidelberg to be assessed?

P. Caspari et al., *At some point there has to be peace and quiet!*,
https://doi.org/10.1007/978-3-658-39785-2_2

- How was H. M.'s membership in AKJP-Heidelberg terminated?
- What network structures existed within the Institute and between the analytical institutes in Heidelberg that prevented the boundary violations from being uncovered for a long time?
- What was the influence of H. M. as a training director on the development of the psychoanalytic identity of the trainees at that time?
- What were the effects of the sexual violence and the work of H. M. at the AKJP-Heidelberg on the Institute and on the psychoanalytic training at the Institute ?
- What were the effects of the sexual violence on the individual groups affected (patients [female and male children and adolescents], training candidates, teaching analysands, staff)?
- What measures have been taken so far to support victims and to prevent further sexual assaults within AKJP-Heidelberg?
- Are there any further indications of cases of sexual violence within AKJP-Heidelberg?

2.2 Advisory Structure

The research was supported by an advisory group, which included representatives of the AKJP-Heidelberg (who work there in various functions) as well as a survivor. The advisory group met four times during the research period. Significant support for the research was provided primarily by the AKJP-Heidelberg office and the ethics officers. For example, they sent the letters with the calls for interview participation to the (former) training candidates, made documentary material accessible and were available at any time for questions or temporal classifications.

The Advisory Group also played an essential role in the planning and implementation of the public calls for participation and the press events organized for this purpose.

Methodology

3

3.1 Access to the Research Field, Data Collection

The main intention of the research working through the H. M. case is a multi-perspective reconstruction of historical facts. Multi-perspective approaches are in a position to reveal contexts of emergence and concealment in relation to institutional violence and to provide explanations as to why cases of sexualised violence in particular remained uncovered for a long time or did not lead to effective institutional reactions that would have ensured the sustainable protection of children and young people and other affected groups.

The study was designed qualitatively. Semi-structured, qualitative interviews and a file and documentary analysis formed the methodological core, supplemented by a literature review.

The file and documentary material came from various sources: On the one hand, archive material of the AKJP-Heidelberg was available to us. This was partly incomplete; for example, minutes of general meetings or letters from professional associations, which were referred to in existing sources, were missing.

On the other hand, we were able to access material that individual members or functionaries of the AKJP-Heidelberg had collected on their own initiative. This includes, among other things, memory protocols and personal records.

Another important source of data are the diaries and memoirs of H. M., which we were able to consult thanks to the permission of his widow. This made many facts from the perpetrator's perspective accessible. The diaries replace an interview with H. M. that was planned but never came about. H. M. died in March 2019.

P. Caspari et al., *At some point there has to be peace and quiet!*,
https://doi.org/10.1007/978-3-658-39785-2_3

We were able to benefit from the preparatory work carried out at the Heidelberg University Hospital, Institute for Psychosocial Prevention, when viewing this biographical material. There, H. M.'s autobiographical bequest was digitized and put into chronological order in preparation for a possible research project.

Due to research ethics and data protection, only those interview partners could be asked directly who are persons of public interest, i.e. who, for example, hold positions in the AKJP-Heidelberg that make it necessary to mention their name publicly (for example, on the homepage) or who were directly connected with commissioning the research project to the IPP Munich. This also applies to experts who are known by name through their publications or their participation in public discourse.

Other key stakeholders and contemporary witnesses were partly approached by the current functionaries of the AKJP-Heidelberg and asked to get in touch with the IPP Munich. The different cohorts of the training candidates of the AKJP-Heidelberg and the IPP-Heidelberg-Mannheim were contacted in three waves by the office of the AKJP-Heidelberg:

- Call 1a: Training candidates of the AKJP-Heidelberg (training years 1975–1995), 60 letters were sent in June 2019,
- Call 1b: Training candidates of the AKJP-Heidelberg (training years 1996–2019), 53 letters were sent in December 2019.
- Call 2: Training candidates of the IPP-Heidelberg-Mannheim (born 1975–1993), about 170 letters were sent in April 2020.

Apart from a few exceptions (scheduling problems, cancellations at short notice), all persons who had responded to the calls were interviewed. Initially, the interviews took place in person, usually in the respective practice rooms of the interviewees or in AKJP-Heidelberg. From spring 2020 onwards, the interviews were conducted by telephone or video, due to the Coronavirus pandemic.

The interviews were semi-structured and problem-centered. The explicit aim was to generate narratives from the interviewees, with corresponding follow-up questions based on the guide. On the one hand, the interviews aimed to provide material for the historical reconstruction of the events in the era of H. M. era, but also to trace the atmosphere in the institute and to give space to personal memories with all their subjective colorations. This allowed for making visible the conditions that made the events possible, as well as the contexts of concealment and disclosure (see Sect. 3.2).

The perspective of the victims is central to the scientific working through the history of sexual boundary violations/sexual violence. A special feature of the events at the AKJP-Heidelberg emerged from the very beginning that those affected were not visible there, that they did not come out publicly as affected persons, except to the contact person at the IPP-Heidelberg-Mannheim at the time. This was initially true for the affected trainees, but also for most of the (former) patients and even more so for children and adolescents who experienced boundary violations by H. M. in the context of second sights or delegation examinations.[1]

In order to be able to reach this group as well, a public call for participation was launched within the framework of a press campaign. For this purpose, two press releases were produced, one by the IPP Munich and one by the AKJP-Heidelberg. The production of the latter and the step towards the public made clear which tense dynamic the Causa H. M. still unfolds in the Institute today when it comes to positioning oneself in relation to its past. This dynamic was discussed and reflected upon in the context of an extraordinary accompanying group meeting moderated by IPP Munich.

The press campaign was ultimately successful. Two articles about the case of H. M. and the scientific inquiry appeared in the regional press:

- "Heidelberg institute wants to reveal family secret" in the Mannheimer Morgen on 02.06.2020 and
- "Institute works through its leader's abuse of power after decades" in Rhein Neckar Zeitung on 10.06.2020.

On the basis of these articles, seven people contacted IPP Munich, including three victims.

However, there were no (former) training candidates among the victims. However, patients from the therapy with H. M. himself or from second sights or examinations in the context of the delegation procedures with him could be interviewed. These interviews finally disproved the long-held narrative that H. M. had never "abused" children or adolescents or that it was only a matter of harmless "playfulness".

A total of 47 interviews were conducted (Table 3.1). Of these, 45 were in-depth, semi-strcutured interviews (duration 90–120 min); in addition, there were two short telephone interviews. Some interview partners also provided us with written material.

Under key stakeholders we subsumed those interview partners who had taken on central functions in AKJP-Heidelberg or IPP-Heidelberg-Mannheim or in the Heidelberg "scene", e.g. as a board member, in another leading position or as a lecturer/supervisor. In this group there is a partial overlap with the group of training

[1] However, until the calls for participation in the context of this study, there had been no active and systematic search for victims.

Table 3.1 Number of interviews by groups. (Own representation)

Group	Number of interviews
Training candidates	25
Experts	3
Key stakeholders	14
Victims	4
Total	**46**

candidates, both from the AKJP-Heidelberg and from the IPP-Heidelberg-Mannheim.

The interviews were recorded, transcribed and analysed using the MAXQDA analysis software. Data collection and data analysis are discussed in detail in the following sections.

3.2 Interleaving of Data Collection and Data Analysis

3.2.1 Theoretical Research Framework

In the context of the research project presented here, a clear differentiation must be made between two different types of results, each based on different research approaches:

1. Results that refer to the proof of facts, namely to the acts of H. M. and the events of unveiling and woking through them. These results, which are based on the study of files, protocols and H. M.'s diary and were supplemented and substantiated by evidence from the interviews, are presented as descriptive findings in Chap. 4.
2. Results that serve to understand the psychological, social and communicative processes underlying the descriptive data collected. Here, above all, the interviews conducted within the framework of the research project function as data sources.

While the results described under (1) primarily required a systematic collection, sorting, contextualizing and relating of information, the generation of the findings characterized under (2) requires a qualitative evaluation strategy, which is described in detail below. It should be noted that the various data sources were repeatedly related to each other in the course of the research process.

Each research field requires its specific pattern of requirements to break down the data obtained. The concept of "Grounded Theory" (Glaser & Strauss, 1998) is often used as a methodological frame of reference for qualitative social research projects. For the analysis of the data obtained on the basis of this paradigm, the program MAXQDA is often used, and it was also applied in the present study. There are a number of theoretically well-founded approaches for the methodological procedure of analysis, such as content analysis (Mayring, 1983, 2015), circular deconstruction (Jaeggi et al., 2004), objective hermeneutics (Oevermann, 1995), the documentary method (Bohnsack, 2000) or qualitative content analysis (Kuckartz, 2012). In our analysis, we draw elements from several of the approaches listed here. In doing so, we were guided above all by the idea that a particular field of research always produces a particular methodology for generating and evaluating data.

The methodology originally developed by Glaser & Strauss in the book Discovery of the Grounded Theory emerged from research on dying people in hospital (Glaser & Strauss, 1967, 2009). Grounded theory is a methodological perspective developed from symbolic interactionism (Blumer, 1973). It does not prescribe rigid procedures, but allows for variably malleable strategies, each producing its own research practices. It is therefore all the more important to be transparent with regard to the description of the methods used in order to enable comprehensibility. Any contradictions found in the data collected must therefore be presented, as must the technique of comparative contrasting of data from different data sources be presented. By identifying the researcher's interpretations as such and relating latent and manifest data to each other, the claim to sufficient validity of the collected findings can be realized. Since qualitative research in this sense refrains from reproducing an objective truth,[2] an open and non-judgmental approach to the research field serves as a criterion for its quality, in addition to the aforementioned transparency with regard to the research method.

Qualitative research is also characterised by an inductive procedure in the different stages of analysis. In the context of an initial evaluation of the collected data, there is a reflexive approach to the research field, whereby thematic areas are initially openly coded by marking certain statements that appear to be particularly relevant. However, the analysis of interview data does not remain purely descriptive and paraphrastic, but is pre-structured by contextual knowledge and the draw-

[2] However, the claim to the reproduction of objective facts is very much realized with regard to the descriptive findings in Chap. 4.

ing on of further sources, which are incorporated into the formation of thematic categories. First, however, certain codes (encryption) are developed within the framework of so-called open coding, whereby commonalities and differences between the interviews are established through permanent comparison. In a further step, codes are combined into categories. The formation of categories thus serves to link the data obtained from the interviews (in the sense of an empirical source) with the increasing contextual knowledge that emerges in the research team during the project. The categories developed from some of the interviews are then used to code the newly collected interviews and make further discriminations and changes to the empiricism-theory linkage (Glaser & Strauss, 1998). Thus, the evaluation is a circular, spiral development of the data material. In a search movement researchers move back and forth between data sources from the research field and the context analysis and exchange their analysis at regular intervals (cf. Caspari, 2012).

In the present research project, these search movements were particularly insightful because the research team had at its disposal three sources of data that were as diverse as they were rich:

- Interviews with stakeholders,
- Protocols and documents
- Diaries

3.2.2 Qualitative Interviews

The chosen qualitative research approach by means of interviews requires some preliminary considerations: What kind of data should be produced? How can data be obtained? How can insights be gained about a case[3]? Starting from anticipations about meaningful case results, it requires considerations about how to "illuminate" a case as comprehensively as possible and in what way a variety of perspectives can be integrated. That is, who and what contributes to adequately describing a case? A case description does not mean a descriptive account of an individual case, but its re-constructive analysis from the data material according to the procedures described above. The representation of the case is subject to a multifaceted transformation process, since one must ultimately choose a selection and thus a reduc-

[3] The definition of "case" is open in qualitative research. Here, it can mean both the "whole" object of study on which a research project focuses, as well as a specific person who "serves as a data source" in the context of an interview.

tion of the data through certain criteria (Merkens, 2003; Rosenthal & Fischer-Rosenthal, 2003).

In the present research field, an interview-based data collection with different participants – contemporary witnesses, victims – seemed appropriate. In an interview situation, two subjects meet to discuss "the case". In doing so, they each have different knowledge and different motivations with regard to the case. However, both "parties" do not know at the beginning of the data collection to what extent the other party is informed and how much knowledge has already been conveyed. This means that on the one hand both are initiates and at the same time ignorants in the field, so that their interaction is also of interest in the context of a subject-oriented approach (Hermanns, 2003). This is especially crucial in the research field studied here, as we interviewed psychoanalysts who are used to asking questions and interpreting interactions due to their professional socialization. The interview situation initially reverses this position, which not infrequently led to initial irritations: Who asks first? How much do I have to talk? How long will the interview take? In addition, some interviewees needed unequivocal reassurance and assertion: Why does the case have to be reopened? Why now of all times? Who has commissioned whom?

In the following example, different situations for information and also misinformation can be seen, which first had to be clarified in the interview with a psychotherapist. It was interesting to ask about the existing subjective hypotheses about how the research assignment came about.

A: I would still be interested in your background now, so that I know (?) are you now permanently employed at the institute, or are you, so to speak, commissioned from somewhere else?

I: Exactly. So there are many permanent employees in the institute. I myself work on a fee basis. I'm a psychological psychotherapist, depth psychology, and I do it because I'm interested and because it's a part-time job at IPP Munich.

A: You are an adult psychotherapist?

I: Exactly.

A: And did I understand that correctly, these are the child analysts who want to work this up?

I: Exactly. The order came from the AKJP (Heidelberg), exactly.

A: The child analysts.

I: Exactly. They have commissioned this.

A: Just so I know when I'm talking to you.

I: Yeah sure.

Many interviews took place in the offices of our interviewees, which also contributed to the above-mentioned reversal of their usual professional situation. Later, due to the pandemic and the subsequent lockdown, interviews were also conducted by video or telephone. It can be assumed that this had an influence on the interactions and thus on the data. Analogous to a psychoanalytic treatment conducted via video, a qualitative interview is also associated with different conversational qualities when conducted via video – as compared to face-to-face contact. However, as the collection of manifest data was also an important part of our research brief, the project also benefited greatly from interviews conducted by telephone or video. However, differences between the interview settings were reflected in the analysis of the data.

But it was not only on the side of the interviewees that a certain caution was recognizable; as researchers ourselves, we also encountered "professional analysts" not without presuppositions. First of all, due to the role of the interviewees, it can be assumed that they have specific knowledge and "tools" with regard to interviewing and reflection. As interviewers, we thus found ourselves in part in a double role as scientists and professional colleagues. The creation of a successful interview situation is incumbent on both parties by showing empathy in order to enable an opening of the interview space in the first place (Hermanns, 2003). This puts the interviewer in a challenging position, as on the one hand s/he has to show understanding for the difficulties of the interview situation, but at the same time s/he has to ask certain questions with regard to results. Hermanns says that the interviewer can also get into a protective attitude towards the interviewee, fearing embarrassment and violations of intimacy and therefore avoiding, for example, inquiries in the case of contradictions (Hermanns, 2003). It is important to reflect on this in advance and to prepare accordingly and to include it in the analysis of the data at the latest.

3.2.3 Hermeneutic Approach

Already during the preparation of the interview guide, certain presuppositions about the acquisition of the data material became clear. For example, we were interested in what motivated the interviewee to participate in the study, what contextual knowledge s/he brings in, and what reflective thoughts s/he has about the case. In addition to this objective information, which is necessary to contextualize the interview and the categories of analysis and to classify what was said, however, latent interview content is also important. Therefore, an open approach beyond the interview guide is additionally required, for example, to enable follow-up questions in case of emerging contradictions.

The first step in the analysis is to allow the interviews to speak for themselves – similar to the countertransference feelings of the analysts. The first sentences, scenes, situations or constellations can be important for the further analysis. These contribute to the initial orientation, but since they are latent information, they must be validated during the analysis and with further data. If they do not find any further points of reference in the analysis, they are dropped. It is interesting, however, that the latent information often emerges again as manifest data in the interview. An example of this would be being late for the interview or forgetting the interview date, which is reflected in confusion about the content or forgetting dates and names in relation to the case being researched. Although missing or fragmentary memories are of course also due to the fact that the era of H. M. was a long time ago, their accumulation nevertheless appeared symptomatic. Confusion about dates (especially times and names) was experienced not only by the interviewees, but also by the research team itself. Time and again, there were ambiguities about when and in what capacity which persons were involved in certain events and facts. These anomalies were, among other things, the subject of discussions about the analysis and the direction of the research process, so that in order to achieve the greatest possible precision of the data, "readjustments" had to be made again and again. Similar to the procedure in Balint groups, we increasingly had the feeling that the case of H. M. with all its ramifications and contradictions was being replayed in our discussions.

Especially in the analysis method of depth hermeneutics, the fact that observable enactments map the latent content of the data finds an explicit consideration (König, 2003). Therefore, parallels between the psychoanalytic approach and the interpretation of qualitative data are often pointed out in qualitative methodology (Devereux, 1984). But there are parallels not only in the analysis of the data, but also in the "getting involved with each other" in the interview. Thus, an analyst should direct all his/her senses to the encounter with the analysand and perceive with equal attention how the conversation and the scene reflect the earlier experience in its specific form (Freud, 1912). In doing so, not only the verbal and factual knowledge is of interest, but also an understanding that goes beyond this is to be intuitively tapped. Accordingly, the researcher as well as the analyst will implicate the material. This entanglement is important because only in this way can an understanding of the retrospectively observed dynamics be made possible. Only by getting involved in the interview situation and thus in a reenactment can a picture of the research object (re)represent itself. However, similar to the analysis, the implication must be understood and interpreted in order to develop explanations and insights on a meta-level. A similar methodological approach is described, for example, by Burka et al. (2019), who investigated the dynamics in a psychoanalytic institute in California in the wake of serious ethical violations by key colleagues: "We offer the collected interview responses not as 'facts' but as the result of conscious and unconscious exchanges that occurred between each participant/interviewer dyad, which were then subjected to analysis" (p. 254). The authors speak here of a two-stage process, whereby the interviewees are first given the opportunity to present their own experiences, while in the second stage it is the task of the researchers to interpret the data collected. Since meanings and interpretations are generated at both stages of this process, the authors refer to the procedure as "double-hermeneutic" (Burka et al., 2019, p. 254).

Thus, the step of looking at and mapping the manifest data in order to mirror other interpretations against it proved to be all the more important for us. For example, by listing the individual boundary violations that can be proven and by presenting the exact analysis of the protocols from that time (cf. Wolff, 2003).

Thus, qualitative analysis always involves a reconstruction of the data obtained, which must continually reassure itself as to what can be found in the data. The movement of induction and deduction ends in an abductive conclusion to which the further procedure is oriented (Dausien, 1995; Reichertz, 2003). This logical conclusion does not emerge somehow, but in the engagement with and through the involvement in the data and the object of research.

Through the precise analysis of the minutes (from general meetings, letters, meetings, …) a documentary reality is established, which could be contrasted with the statements made in the interviews. What is exciting about this process, which is staggered in time and intertwined through the confrontation with the present-day interview data, is that one can increasingly recognize persons and their entanglements in the aftermath. As a result, insights are generated by both what is said and what is not said. Through the interlaced analysis of the data sources, which at times takes on the character of detective reconstructions, gaps in information and knowledge are gradually filled in. In this way, it also becomes clear in the course of the research process that some interviewees, consciously aware of these gaps, did not disclose certain information, so that the analysis is also directed at the motivations associated with that behavior. Against the background that not all interviewees are equally informed, our task also consisted of assigning them as precisely as possible to specific periods and contexts (e.g. AKJP-Heidelberg or IPP-Heidelberg-Mannheim, year of training, etc.…). For this purpose, both the protocols and diaries served as well as corresponding inquiries in the interviews. Although the protocols are "closer to the events" than the actual interviews and thus convey a conclusive temporal orientation, these data sources also ultimately reflect a construction of these events, which must be deconstructed accordingly (Wolff, 2003).

Such deconstructions require above all a separation of content, form and interpretation.

When we interpret data retrospectively, the question of the contemporary history of the 1970s and 1980s and the discourse knowledge about sexual abuse available at that time also plays a role. The historical background of the arguments about sexual abuse in psychotherapy and especially in psychoanalysis also serves as an interpretive template and provides further framing. Therefore, it was important not only to interview contemporary witnesses who directly contributed to this historical process, but also to undertake an extensive analysis of contemporary publications on this topic.

3.2.4 Validation of Interview Data: The Narrative Approach

The motivation reported by the respective interviewees to participate in the study often forms a level of reflection to which further statements from an interview are related. This applies not only to the group of interviewees who were rather critical of the project of working through the history, but also to those who were in favour of the study. Among other things, statements that refer to actual or presumed knowledge or to the alleged lack of knowledge can be classified on this level of reflection. The following two quotes from the interview with a psychotherapist are examples of frequently occurring narratives of non-knowledge or assumed knowledge.

> I: And the son, he was H. M.'s son.
> A: Yes. He looked a lot like him too, he couldn't deny his father. So (laughs) he looked very much like him.
> I: But who was the mother? Did you know that?
> A: Mother, I have no idea. I didn't know, there wasn't one, so at least I wasn't aware of one.
> Well they could have, they could have stopped this! They knew, they knew what was going on! They did – that's what they said, H. M. didn't deny the child he had there, who was jumping around at the institute. So it was known! They all did nothing – not just nothing.

Here, for the analysis one could ask: Who may have known what? Why did the interviewee not know anything, but is sure that others knew something? Thus, the task arises here to analyse the interview in more detail and to relate it to further manifest data from other interviews. Therefore, it is important to include a certain number of interview partners in order to achieve the necessary breadth of information. However, the selection of the interview partners was not arbitrary, but hypothesis-driven in the sense of "theoretical sampling" (Glaser, 1978). This is connected with the question, which always has to be asked anew, which perspectives and contemporary witnesses can still be expected to provide meaningful information for the case under investigation. In the present field of investigation, it was noticeable that there were many cross-references by the interviewees to possible persons in the know and also those affected, who, however, did not participate in an interview. Thus, one always had the feeling that there was a web of shadow interviewees and contextual knowledge buzzing in the orbit of the study, but that it could not be translated into manifest data. This observation must also be included in the analysis or already represents an important result.

In addition to the approach of "Grounded Theory", which originates from the tradition of symbolic interactionism and addresses the external perspective of the analysis as an action-theoretical meta-level, the internal perspective of the interviewees in the present field of investigation can be captured through the analysis of narratives. This is not only about descriptions of such perspectives, but also about their representations. The interviewee appears both as a first-person narrator and as a first-person figure who relates to the reported case. The development of a narrative takes place within the framework of the production of a we-reality in which the listener functions as a point of reflection and part of the story. Particular attention is paid to the time horizon of an interview, as both the current present and the retrospective view of the past and expectations with regard to a future perspective are inquired about (Rosenthal & Fischer-Rosenthal, 2003). In the present case, this is particularly exciting, as the research was initiated as a result of the court case against H. M. and the publication of the article in the "ZEIT". Both events led to strong reactions in the research field, not least because, on the one hand, they made information about the past available, but on the other hand, they also revealed many unanswered questions. All in all, a time span of 27 years after the first serious disclosure of the assaults represents a rather extensive, but by no means exceptional, investigative perspective for an external project of working through the history. For the analysis, narratives from the present-day perspective, in which earlier facts are interpreted on the basis of current events and discourses, represent the central focal point. The narrative based on recollections always takes place with recourse to an immediate evaluation of the present situation and with an orientation to what has been told could mean for the future. In qualitative social research, narration is considered a "key discipline of cultural studies" (Köhle & Koerfer, 2011; Vogd, 2005), but at the same time it comes under criticism for being (rightly?) sceptical of the narrated and the narrator. Rosenthal and Fischer-Rosenthal, for example, regard their studies and evaluations of narrated life stories as hypothetical in principle.

This means that hypotheses are addressed to the material on the basis of the analysis of individual parts of the conversation, which can only be confirmed or refuted within the text and its narrative structure (Rosenthal, 1987; Rosenthal & Fischer-Rosenthal, 2003). Here is an example from an interview with a psychotherapist in the context of our study:

I: And why didn't anyone say anything?
A: Ah, many people have said something. That was also a topic at the conferences, at the VAKJP; and: Scandal! and so on. And last year I got a letter from X, where he talks about the cover-up system, a "notorious cover-up system" here in Heidelberg, right, and there was an incredibly hurtful and angry …, an angry attack also on me. And the Y then tried to explain that a bit, why the X is so hurtful, right? Because they were – that was the powerlessness, so it was yes … I mean, the professional association was powerless, there was no protocol, right? to withdraw that from him. Yes? Because …
I: You still have to explain that to me. Why was there no protocol if someone so …
A: There was no proof, right? There was some …
I: So now we leave the children's matters out of it: But now, as far as the abstinence violation is concerned, that was almost on record here.
A: Yes, that …
I: Should this have been charged from within the institute, or should it have been charged and we should have said: We can prove that he had sexual relations with at least five analysands? The number is arbitrary now, but …
A: Yes, it was clear about the children (…), because they had …
I: He fathered children twice, but in retrospect married only once.
A: But in the field of children's therapy and diagnostics, the encroachment in diagnostics, yes?, we could only …
I: Only indirectly infer it.
A: Indirectly, yes, indirectly. So we may have been cowardly too, yes?, we may have been fearful too. That's what I would say, yeah. And that's the way it is: You don't want to have to deal with this shit all the time, right?

In this section of the interview, the ambivalence or rather the juxtaposition of knowing and not knowing, of doing and refraining, of feasibility and powerlessness is formulated. In the narration and formulation of the "facts" as they are perceived, they increasingly become a reality in the interview, but at the same time they always already were. However, through the updating in the research interview secured by audio recording, this narrative can also have implications for the future. In the analysis of narratives, breaks and interruptions in the narrative flow are also of interest, as they can provide indications of blocking (Rosenthal, 1987). In the excerpt of conversation here, one can surmise that the interviewee is asking himself why more has not been done and what it means when he articulates exactly this in the context of the interview. By empathically going along with the interview situation, the interviewer signals that, on the one hand, he can understand that it was difficult to take action, but on the other hand, he also expresses surprise that existing factual knowledge at the time was insufficiently acknowledged. The questions that arise in this sequence cannot be answered within the framework of this interview alone, but only by consulting other interviewees and data. The interviewee gives the impression that the question of inadequate interventions in the past is either only now imposing itself on him in all clarity or he is afraid of burdening himself or others too much if he names the facts too precisely. Accordingly, he seems receptive to the justification offered to him by the interviewer that one could only indirectly conclude that there had been assaults against children, so that he is able to find a way out of what is for him a difficult section of the conversation.

However, the explanatory value of this line of argument is only provisional, since the fundamental question remains open as to why efforts to clarify the situation at the time (e.g. with the help of the review of files) regularly came to nothing:

> I: You just had a look and you found what you were looking for. So you have …
> A: Let's put it this way, you would have to take a closer look: Who was on the board at that time? (…) Or what were the leading figures? Or so. So maybe you could also look a little bit more. I think that has a lot to do with the A. A., that there was no impetus that would have perhaps also promoted us: Continue there. Yes? Or we have to uncover that or something. But of course there was always a brake in it, yes? That's what I would say.
> I: So in retrospect, yes.
> A: I didn't perceive it that way back then. And I mean, we are also, in that respect, pfff … As far as such things are concerned, one is quite happy to get out of the thing again, isn't it? Or you like to deny it again or let it rest a bit or something. Yes? Yes, that's true. We haven't followed it up in detail. So that would certainly be an interesting conversation with those who were involved at the time, to reflect on how it actually went.

The formulated contradiction of investigating on the one hand, but always getting stuck and not doing anything further on the other, is revealed again. This is also evident in the language style of the interview. Not only the interviewee repeatedly breaks off his sentences, but also the interviewer interrupts the narrative flow, as if past actions and thoughts were mirrored as a structural equation in the formulation of the present interlocutors.

From today's perspective, the question arises as to why more consistent action was not taken at that time. In the same way, however, it can be asked what prompted the Institute to bring the case of H. M. to the surface again and again, although it was in a certain sense closed. Something obviously could not come to rest.

This brief example was intended to illustrate how narratives can be methodically opened up and data interpreted. Qualitative social research always considers the narrative on a symbolic level of the event. It is through the narrative and its structure that the case reveals itself as that which constitutes the research field.

Here, too, there is a parallel to the practice of psychoanalysis, which deals with the narratives of patients and their meaning and transforms them into interpretations. Strictly speaking, one could fundamentally doubt the empirical "veracity" of qualitative interview data collected in the social sciences. But similar to psychoanalysis, the dialogue within the interview represents a particularly meaningful access to knowledge in a subject-oriented field. The narrative in which the story is verbalized and in which we verbalize and formulate ourselves in the story is what creates cognition.

4 Descriptive Findings as a Frame of Reference

4.1 Assaults, Boundary Violations, Sexual Violence: Findings on the Crimes of H. M

The following is a compilation of sexual assaults committed by H. M. as well as sexual relations of H. M. in the context of his activities at the AKJP-Heidelberg and at the IPP-Heidelberg-Mannheim. As described above, the following data sources serve as the basis for this information:

- oral and written reports from victims;
- oral and written reports, especially from former employees and managers of the Children's Institute and the Adult Institute (mainly information from our qualitative interviews);
- Files and minutes from the AKJP-Heidelberg; minutes from the IPP-Heidelberg-Mannheim; (diary entries by H. M.).

Only those hints that can be regarded as highly probable have been included in the listing. This is not to be understood in the sense of a judicial conclusiveness, but as the result of thorough checks of the above-mentioned sources, which led to the assessment that the corresponding information can be considered sufficiently plausible. This also implies that some indications on the basis of secondary sources (indications of third parties, which were communicated to us by our interviewpartners) were taken into account.

Following the rather cursory list of reported sexual boundary violations and sexual relations, some information is given in an overview-like mention to, in our

P. Caspari et al., *At some point there has to be peace and quiet!*,
https://doi.org/10.1007/978-3-658-39785-2_4

view, provide an important contextualization of the information classified as secure.

Demonstrable sexual boundary violations and sexual relations of H. M. in the context of the two training institutes AKJP-Heidelberg and IPP-Heidelberg-Mannheim:

1. In relation to a celebration on the occasion of H. M.'s appointment as head of the institute, which takes place about a year after he began his work at AKJP-Heidelberg (1975), a "dodgy" and "encroaching" atmosphere is reported. The atmosphere between H. M. and some training candidates is described as inappropriate in the sense of unclear demarcations.
2. Around 1976, H. M. has a sexual relationship with a training candidate who is training both at the Adult Institute and – temporarily – at the Children's Institute.
3. At an unspecified time in the years 1975–1977, a child patient (boy of elementary school age) is asked by H. M. to strip naked as part of his second sight.
4. In 1976, during a psychotherapeutic session, H. M. tells a 15-year-old female patient that she should not be afraid of her first sexual contact. He offers to show her how it is done. In response to her irritated inquiry as to what he specifically meant by this, he replies that he can do it with her here (in the treatment room). In the following sessions he repeatedly brings up this subject of his own accord and several times offers to go away with her (by train). He makes further sexual advances towards her. He also touches her breasts.
5. In 1977 or 1978 H. M. asks a 14 or 15 year old female patient during a psychotherapeutic session whether she would sometimes look at herself naked in the mirror. He also inquires of her whether she would sometimes caress herself when she was naked, including in the genital area. H. M. asks these questions despite clear discomfort on the part of the patient. As she continues, H. M. leans far forward and asks in a gentle voice, "How would it be if I took you in my arms and caressed you? Would you like that?" This leads to further serious stress reactions on the part of the patient.
6. In 1979, H. M. begins a sexual relationship with the 18-year-old R. R. The latter had been admitted as a patient by H. M. when she was 16 years old. The sexual relationship presumably begins after the completion of therapy. At the age of 19 Ms. R. gives birth to a boy. H. M. is the father of this child.
7. On an unspecified date in the late 1970s/early 1980s, a boy was touched or indecently touched by H. M. on several occasions in the course of psychotherapeutic treatment.

8. On an unspecified date (presumably in the 1970s) H. M. touches the breast of a 14-year-old female patient in the course of a second sight, she visits the Children's Institute due to sexual assaults she has suffered herself. He commits this act under the pretext of wanting to re-enact the sexual assault described by the teenager.
9. In the years 1979–1981 (or 1980–1982) H. M., as head of the institute, has a sexual relationship with the training candidate D. T. The contact with Ms. T. continues at least until 1990, although it is unclear whether sexual encounters still occur during this period. During her relationship with H. M., Ms. T. is married. Among other things, she asks a fellow trainee to put her apartment at her disposal for a few days so that she can meet H. M. there undisturbed.
10. In 1982 H. M., in his function as a teaching analyst (at the IPP-Heidelberg-Mannheim), begins a sexual relationship with the married teaching analyst B. U. This relationship lasts until 1990. Although she has not yet completed her training, H. M. helps Mrs. U. to become a lecturer at the AKJP-Heidelberg.
11. During an indeterminable period of time, H. M. always grabs a trainee candidate who is in supervision with him around the waist as a greeting, guides her into the treatment room and frequently touches her thigh during the sessions.
12. Around the mid-1980s, a patient of about 14/15 years of age is presented to H. M. for a second sight. H. M. "plays" with the teenager's penis during the examination.
13. In 1986 or 1987 a girl of about 10 or 11 years is referred to the AKJP-Heidelberg with a suspected post-traumatic stress disorder. In the initial interview H. M. asks her unpleasant questions about sexuality (e.g. how she feels about naked men, whether she already has a developing breast) and repeatedly probes her about this. He makes her do exercises which, in retrospect, give her the impression that he wanted to see her breasts. He also touches her in an uncomfortable way. She refuses further appointments.
14. In November 1988, H. M. begins a sexual relationship with his 18-year-old patient J. E. This relationship lasts for over a year (approximately until January 1990).

(There are different statements about the age of the patient: There is also talk that she was only 15 or 16 years old at the beginning of the relationship with H. M.).

15. In 1989, a 7-year-old patient has to take off his pants in front of H. M., which allows H. M. to look at the boy's penis.
16. H. M. has had sexual contacts with A. A. since 1989 at the latest. A. (according to assumptions, however, these sexual contacts also existed much earlier,

namely already at the time of her training at AKJP-Heidelberg). At this time A. A. is a member of the board of AKJP-Heidelberg. She completed her training as a child and adolescent psychotherapist at AKJP-Heidelberg in 1978–1983, worked there as a lecturer and was elected to the board of the institute in 1987. It is unclear how long there is sexual contact between H. M. and A. A. after 1990. A. A. is married and has a daughter. The latter is friends with E. M. in her adolescence. In about 1987, E. M. lives with the A. family for about a year.

17. Since 1988 at the latest (but presumably earlier), H. M. has had a sexual relationship with the married V. G. It is unclear whether she is a trainee or a patient.
18. In 1989, already at the beginning of the psychotherapeutic treatment of a 20-year-old female patient, sexual assaults (looks at the breasts) were committed by H. M. The psychotherapist questioned the young woman forcefully and in detail about the massive sexual violence experiences she had suffered at the hands of her foster father. The patient has the impression that H. M. "gets excited" by these descriptions.
19. In 1989 or 1990 H. M. rubs the penis of the 4-year-old patient T. L. who is lying on the examination couch in the treatment room. H. M. says to the boy that he could do this more often in the future.
20. At an unspecified time (late 1980s/early 1990s), H. M. "plays" with the penis of a patient (probably of elementary school age).
21. At the beginning of 1990, H. M. begins a sexual relationship with his 21-year-old patient E. M. (see case 18). This relationship resulted in a daughter in 1991 (born 07.07.1991). When E. M. was pregnant with the second daughter, H. M. and E. M. get married on 18.03.1993. The second daughter is born on 03.07.1993. The couple separated in 2016.
22. At least since the early 1990s, H. M. has had a sexual relationship with his teaching analyst, I. O.
23. From 1992 onwards, four or five women reported to a director of the IPP-Heidelberg-Mannheim that they had been sexually assaulted by or had sexual relations with H. M. in the course of teaching analyses or supervision. Among them are the cases documented under points 10 and 22. No information can be given about the two or three other cases.
24. At a point in time that cannot be determined more precisely (presumably in the early 1990s), H. M. sexually assaults a pair of brothers (presumably of primary school age) during an initial assessment.
25. At an unspecified point in time, a 5–6 year old patient has to "get naked" in the context of second sight with H. M.. H. M. touched the boy's penis.

26. On an unspecified date, an 8-year-old girl refuses further appointments with H. M. on the grounds, expressed to her mother, that it is "piggy" with him.
27. In 1994, during an open-house day, parents complain to a therapist of the educational counselling center Ebersbach (and former training candidate at the AKJP-Heidelberg) about boundary violations committed against their children at the AKJP-Heidelberg. Even if this is not explicitly mentioned, it can be assumed that the incriminated assaults were carried out by H. M.. It is unclear how many children were affected and when the acts in question were committed.

The following incidents refer to the time when H. M. was no longer working at AKJP-Heidelberg, but had his own practice in Seckach:

28. Probably in the year 1994 H. M. (presumably in the context of a second sight) lets a boy show him his genitals. H. M. inquires from the boy about his masturbation practices and fantasies and masturbates him.
29. Probably in 1995 H. M. asks a patient of about 9 years in the course of a second sight whether the breast of her older sister was already growing and whether her nipple was becoming firm.
30. 1996 In his practice in Seckach H. M. touches a 9-year-old patient between his legs (or in his trousers). For this reason, a preliminary investigation is initiated against H. M., but remains without consequences.
31. Approximately in 1996, a female patient of H. M. is led by him into his bedroom.
32. In 2016, H. M. commits sexual abuse against his 4-year-old granddaughter. In the subsequent court proceedings, he is proven to have committed 11 offences against his granddaughter that meet these criteria. (Further indications of sexual violence within the family are not the subject of the present investigation).

It should be noted that many descriptions are very similar with regard to sexual assaults against boys in the context of second sights. Since these cases were carefully reconstructed, duplications are excluded.

In the following, some information is listed that we classified as (1) not sufficiently substantiated, (2) as minor, (3) as a generalized assessment, (4) as difficult to assign, or (5) as supplementary information to the listing above. However, these references are suitable for completing the picture that can be made of psychotherapist H. M.'s handling of boundaries and of the requirement of abstinence: (A separate section is devoted to non-sexual boundary violations below).

- In 1976, H. M. reported in a medical history record about a boy of just under 9 years of age who "immediately got an erection" during the examination, which – according to H. M. – "is very typical in my experience with day-wetting". According to the report, the boy also described during the examination that he masturbated in the evenings.
- In a second sight record from 1985, H. M. reported in relation to the examination of an 8-year-old boy that in this boy – "as in most of the enuretics I have examined" – an erection was induced by palpation of the abdomen.
- In 1985, H. M. documents in a second sight record that he asked a boy of just under 10 years of age whether he sometimes had a stiffening of the limbs. In the further course he describes reactions of both the boy and the mother to this topic, which express recognizably strong feelings of shame, but which H. M. apparently ignores.
- On an unspecified date, criminal investigations are carried out against H. M. on suspicion of possessing "child pornographic" material. The proceedings are discontinued.

For the overall assessment of the sexual boundary violations against children described here and above, it is important to note that several children are known to have been extraordinarily irritated by H. M.'s behavior, to have strictly refused further appointments with H. M., and in some cases to have suffered long-lasting stress. This information is of particular importance because it does not allow a classification of H. M.'s behaviour as a "normal paediatric examination" under any circumstances. The boys and girls felt ashamed, insecure and threatened by the doctor's transgressions. It should be added that H. M. states in a diary note in 2016 that "during physical examinations of boys at the institute, he [was] only interested in those who spontaneously had an erection when undressing. I waited for this 'signal', then examined, then possibly felt the erection again and the 'ritual' was over."

- At the beginning of 1990, H. M. felt very strongly attracted to a young female patient named K.. It cannot be ascertained whether sexual acts took place with her.
- There is no evidence of any case in which H. M. committed sexual boundary violations against mothers of child patients. Only "strange" statements are reported in the context of case discussions, in which H. M. described certain mothers as "sexually needy". There is, however, one passage in the diary in which H. M. shows great interest in the mother of a patient. He tries to go on a

date with her. However, the rendezvous does not take place. Thereupon H. M. refers the daughter to a colleague.

- At an unspecified time, H. M. told the institute secretary that he would like to have children with her.
- A supervisee of H. M. who had probably done her training at the Adult Institute later told a colleague that H. M. had not committed any sexual assaults against her in the supervisions, "but that she could understand how that went."
- One interviewee reported that H. M. grabbed her brooch pinned at chest level during a supervision session.
- Another interviewee describes H. M.'s aloof behaviour during her job interview.
- In at least one case, it is known that rape by H. M. occurred in the context of a sexual relationship with a female patient.
- It is known about the time after leaving the AKJP Institute Heidelberg in 1993 that H. M. went out to eat with female patients whom he treated in his practice, visited them at home and gave them presents. In one case he had a suit made for him by a patient.
- Current patients of a clinic report that they were victims of H. M. (There are no time details or information as to whether they were affected by H. M.'s assaults as children, adolescents or adults).
- A child and adolescent psychotherapist reported "quite a lot of complaints from patients about H. M." as recently as circa 2016/2017.

With regard to many of the statements made here, it should be noted that a clear assignment of the victims of the boundary violations to the AKJP-Heidelberg on the one hand or to the IPP-Heidelberg-Mannheim on the other appears to be very difficult. In most cases (from secondary sources) there is talk of "training candidates", "teaching analysands", "supervisors" or "colleagues" who were affected by H. M.'s boundary violations. In the overall view of all the information, however, there is no doubt that H. M. committed sexual boundary violations against training candidates or had sexual relations with training candidates or colleagues both at the AKJP-Heidelberg and in the context of his activities at the IPP-Heidelberg-Mannheim. If one combines the information from H. M.'s diary, according to which he had sexual relations with more than 50 women, with his confession, also formulated in his diary, that his social relations were almost exclusively limited to training candidates, patients and colleagues, then cautious hypotheses about the extent of victimization in the context of the psychotherapeutic training institutes in Berlin and Heidelberg could be derived from this.

The data collected and presented here suggest the assumption of an extensive unreported number of sexual boundary violations committed by H. M. against children, adolescents, training candidates, teaching analysts, co-workers, supervisees and adult patients. The more than 30 offences described above are therefore with some certainty only the tip of an iceberg of boundary violations and assaults of which we are not aware. This assumption initially refers to children and adolescents who were presented to H. M. for a second sight or for therapy. It can be assumed that by far not all children and adolescents who were shamed, harassed and touched by the doctor in the examination room confided in their parents. Moreover, certainly not all of the related information that parents have received from their children has been communicated to others. The investigative practices of H. M. that have become known seem to follow a pattern that, while it cannot be generalized without qualification to all sessions conducted by him, does not, on the other hand, appear to be at all random or even "unintentional". Regardless of the underlying motivations of the doctor, there was undoubtedly a disposition on his part to accept feelings of shame and fear experienced by the children he examined, and even to deliberately bring them about. The information we know about boundary violations against adolescent girls is unequivocal. Also in this age group the threshold for the communication of suffered sexual boundary violations is to be regarded as very high, so that only a fraction of the probably common repertoire of invasive questioning, shaming and touching of the attending therapist H. M. should be known to us. The sheer fact that H. M. diagnosed and treated children and adolescents over many decades, and that cases have demonstrably come to light over the entire period of investigation considered here, makes it seem likely that over the course of at least 40 years a very large number of girls and boys had to endure sexual boundary violations by H. M. of varying intensity and frequency. Even if it is not possible to make a serious extrapolation in this regard, it can be considered certain that all children and adolescents who presented to H. M. over the decades were at risk of suffering sexual boundary violations or assaults in the context of treatment, since there is no doubt about the doctor's willingness to commit such acts.

The cases of R. R., E. M. and J. E. make it clear that H. M. sought sexual contacts and relationships with young female patients who had just become adults. The pregnancies of two of these young women led to a partial elucidation of a possibly larger dark figure in relation to this group of people, without leading to the averting of still existing dangers.

With regard to his functions as head of the institute, teaching analyst and supervisor, it can be assumed that H. M. was fundamentally prepared to sexualize such professional settings intentionally, to commit boundary violations and to initiate long-term sexual relationships. From our interviews we know that such offences did not occur in every case, but this does not change the fact that corresponding dangers must be assumed on a regular basis. The spectrum of offenses here ranges from seemingly random touching to "irritating" remarks, suggestive glances, and the unmistakable sexualization of professional settings, sexual acts, and long-term sexual relationships. In view of the important obstacles to detection described in detail below, it must also be assumed that there is a considerable number of unreported cases with regard to such sexual boundary violations in professional settings.

It can be seen from the above list that there were temporal overlaps between boundary violations, assaults and sexual relationships towards different groups of people. This also indicates that H. M. was in principle always willing to initiate constellations of examination, treatment and relationships in which girls, boys and women could potentially be seriously harmed.

4.2 Potentials for Disclosure and Attempts of Inquiry

The following remarks on attempts of disclosure and inquiry are initially mainly descriptive. Thus, it is primarily a matter of a description of what was done or omitted from different sides in relation to a possible disclosure or reflexive processing of H. M.'s deeds. This list forms an empirical basis, so to speak, for the analyses and discussions that follow. However, two preliminary remarks seem appropriate at this point:

1. The distinction between disclosure and inquiry is not a sharp one. A more detailed conceptual discussion will show that these are interlocking processes that are subject to a mutually stimulating dynamic. Nevertheless, for the sake of clarity at the descriptive level discussed here, a differentiation between disclosure and inquiry seems useful to us.
2. The disclosure and inquiry phenomena described here follow a logic that we have described elsewhere as an iterative sequence of latent processes and manifest index events (Caspari 2021a; Mosser & Hackenschmied, 2018). This points to the fact that the situations and constellations listed largely defy isolated consideration and therefore only become understandable against the background of a complex dynamic of processes. Precisely because of this complexity, however, an introductory condensed overview seems appropriate to us, as it provides a stable frame of reference for the analyses that follow.

4.3 Potential for Disclosure: Initiatives and Omissions in Relation to Possible Disclosures

We choose the term "disclosure potentials" here in order to capture disclosure attempts and omissions in equal measure. We are primarily concerned here with the depiction of social interactions that were suitable for transforming sexual violence and damaging relationship constellations from the realm of the microcosm of the intimate relationship or the perpetrator-victim dyad into an arena of social (or partially public) discussion. Since the situations listed often refer to the boundary violations described above, corresponding references are inserted in brackets in each case.

1. H. M. has documented his examination practices and observations in the context of second sights of child patients in several records. There are a number of such protocols from the 1970s onwards, which reveal shameful physical examinations of boys. It can be assumed that these protocols were written by typists and read by the attending child and adolescent psychotherapists (some of whom were also training candidates at the AKJP-Heidelberg). To our knowledge, there was no critical discussion of the examination practices described by H. M. or corresponding communication to other people. It can be assumed that such protocols were written again and again over several decades without anyone taking offence.
2. As early as the 1970s it was known among female trainees at the AKJP-Heidelberg that colleagues were "hit on" by H. M. during supervision sessions.
3. In the mid-1970s, a boy of primary school age tells his mother on the way home after an examination by H. M. that the doctor had asked him to strip naked. After that, there is a maximum of one more examination with H. M. (see case 3).
4. In about 1976 or 1977, at least two women who applied to the AKJP-Heidelberg as training candidates were aware that H. M. had a sexual relationship with a training candidate (at the IPP-Heidelberg-Mannheim and at the AKJP-Heidelberg) (see case 2).
5. At the end of the 1970s a (married) training candidate at the AKJP-Heidelberg is in a relationship with H. M.. This colleague speaks openly about this relationship with other training candidates. In one case she asks a fellow student to let her have her apartment for a few days so that she can spend time there with H. M. undisturbed. Photos of at least one joint trip of H. M. with the

trainee candidate who was in a relationship with him are available at the institute (see case 9).

6. It is known among the training candidates at the AKJP-Heidelberg that a fellow student has had a relationship with the lecturer Dr. M. during her entire training period. This is also dealt with openly.
7. A few contemporary witnesses who did their training at the AKJP-Heidelberg in the 1980s say in the course of our interviews that they noticed that "something was always going on" between H. M. and individual training candidates. It could not be overlooked that certain training candidates were "fascinated" by H. M., "followed him" or were "very close to him". Rumours circulated according to which the willingness to enter into an intimate relationship with H. M. was associated with advantages for the course of the training. His habitus towards individual female trainees is characterized by a contemporary witness as "very physical".
8. According to our data, many people at the AKJP-Heidelberg and at the IPP-Heidelberg-Mannheim were probably aware of the fact that H. M. shifted contacts with both training candidates (and explicitly also to teaching analysands) and patients to outside the professional context. There was talk of meeting H. M. in a wine bar or café if there was something to discuss with him or – even more drastically – "it is best to take the bed sheet with you when you lie down on his couch" (this was also known at IPP-Heidelberg-Mannheim). There are also reports of sauna sessions with female colleagues.
9. There are various reports of institute parties at which, according to the perception of some of those present, an inappropriate closeness between H. M. and individual training candidates became apparent.
10. From 1982 H. M. had a relationship with a training analysand (at the IPP-Heidelberg-Mannheim). In the course of the 1980s he got her a lectureship at the AKJP-Heidelberg. Around 1987 a fellow student at the IPP-Heidelberg-Mannheim observes how this student leaves the house in which H. M. lives in the early morning. Alarmed by this, she tells this incident to her teaching analyst, who, however, does not react. In leading committees of the IPP-Heidelberg-Mannheim it becomes known that H. M. had arranged for his training analysand to work as a lecturer at the AKJP-Heidelberg. This, however, is not problematized. Among the training candidates the relationship between H. M. and the (married) woman working as a lecturer is well known, as both parties involved make no secret of it. From about the end of the 1980s, pictures of joint trips (e.g. to Yemen) hang on walls of the institute. It is known to practically everyone that the travel companion is a training analysand. The

secretary actively draws the attention of training candidates and staff to holiday pictures of the two (see case 10).

11. Around the mid-1980s, a training candidate at the AKJP-Heidelberg tells her teaching analyst that a patient of about 14/15 years came to her session crying because H. M. had been playing with his penis in the context of a second sight (see case 12).
12. Around 1986/1987 a patient of about 10 or 11 years reports to her mother about boundary violating examination practices of H. M. No further appointments with H. M. take place (see case 13).
13. Around the mid-1980s, a patient reports to her psychotherapist that it is known in the "whole district" where she lives and where the AKJP-Heidelberg is also located that H. M. sleeps with his female patients. The psychotherapist casually confronts H. M. with this information, which H. M. dismisses with an indifferent reaction. No further efforts are made to clarify the situation.
14. In February 1989 a 7-year-old boy approaches his mother with the information that he had had to take off his trousers during an examination by H. M., whereupon H. M. had looked at his penis. The mother considers approaching H. M. about this, as her son appears to be very distressed as a result. However, she refrains from doing so (see case 15).
15. H. M.'s son is born in 1980. The mother is a former patient of H. M. and is 19 years old at the time of birth. This circumstance is known to several people in the institute and its environment. H. M. himself proudly announces the birth of his son at the Institute. In the course of the 1980s he is frequently visited by his son (and his mother) in the institute rooms of the AKJP-Heidelberg. Over the years, the secretary repeatedly tells the AKJP-Heidelberg about the relationship from which the child was born. It is not known that this circumstance was discussed critically and in detail with staff members or training candidates at the AKJP-Heidelberg (see case 6). H. M. noted in his diary "…because I, blinded by my fatherly pride, reported the birth of [name of son] myself at the institute, and this news spread like wildfire over all the couches on which my training candidates lay with all the teaching analysts in Heidelberg".
16. At an unspecified time (late 1980s/early 1990s), a boy tells his mother that H. M. played with the boy's penis during an examination after he had asked the mother to leave the examination room. The boy talks about this incident more often, but the mother does not take it seriously (see case 20).
17. At the beginning of 1990 H. M. begins a sexual relationship with a 21-year-old female patient. This patient is friends with the daughter of the head of the AKJP-Heidelberg, A. A.. About 1 or 2 years before, the patient even lived with the A. family for a period of about 1 year. The patient was a very stressed

young woman who had had some severely traumatising experiences in various youth welfare services. There was also a sexual relationship between H. M. and Ms. A. A. during this time (see case 21).

18. At an unspecified point in time (presumably in the early 1990s), H. M. sexually assaults a pair of brothers (presumably of primary school age) during an initial appointment. The boys come home crying and beg their mother never to have to go to an appointment with H. M. again. However, they say nothing about sexual assaults. They later confide in a clergyman about this (see case 24).
19. On the occasion of H. M.'s 60th birthday in July 1992, Dr. M. P. congratulated the jubilarian on the birth of his daughter in a speech at a larger event. The child is 1 year old at this time. Many participants in the event know that this child was the result of a connection between H. M. and a very young (former) patient (see case 21).
20. In temporal proximity to this celebration, a former training candidate and still associated with the AKJP-Heidelberg psychotherapist is informed by a friend that she had presented her son at the Institute at the age of 5 or 6 and that he had had to strip naked during the second sight with H. M. and that the latter had touched his penis (see case 25).
21. In 1992 at the latest, the Youth Welfare Office in Heidelberg became aware of the relationship between H. M. and his (former) patient, who was 37 years younger, which was apparently regarded as problematic. This was presumably also because the young woman had been cared for in the course of her biography in several youth welfare services. There are indications that the Youth Welfare Office discussed the case with the IPP-Heidelberg-Mannheim (see case 21).
22. In 1992 a patient reports to her psychotherapist at the end of the very last therapy session that her son, who is now an adult, had recently confided in her that he had been "indecently touched several times" by H. M. in the course of examinations about 10–15 years ago. The patient does not comply with the psychotherapist's request to be released from her duty of confidentiality. As various accusations against H. M. become public immediately afterwards, the psychotherapist does not take any further action (see case 7).
23. At the end of November 1992 the chairman of the IPP-Heidelberg-Mannheim becomes aware (probably through the Youth Welfare Office) of H. M.'s relation with his (former) patient. An extraordinary general meeting is called for February 1993 in order to expel H. M. from the IPP-Heidelberg-Mannheim (see case 21). From December 1992 onwards, several women contact a board member of the IPP-Heidelberg-Mannheim and report serious abstinence viola-

tions by H. M., mainly in the context of teaching analyses (in total, there are about four or five women who – at times that cannot be reconstructed exactly – contact the board member with corresponding information) (see cases 10 and 22). The contact person, who also works as a lecturer at the AKJP-Heidelberg, carries this information to the board of the IPP-Heidelberg-Mannheim, taking into account the anonymity of the women concerned. At this point, for the first time, there is a fundamental discussion of H. M.'s boundary violations and the threat of consequences.

24. In January 1993 the chairman of the IPP-Heidelberg-Mannheim informs the chairman and the legal adviser of the DGPT about the planned expulsion of H. M. and the corresponding reasons. H. M. resigns his membership in the IPP-Heidelberg-Mannheim in January. He had already been relieved of his functions in the IPP Heidelberg-Mannheim in December 1992. The Association of Statutory Health Insurance Physicians (KV) is also informed that H. M. is no longer active at the IPP-Heidelberg-Mannheim.
25. At the end of January 1993, members of the supporting association of the AKJP-Heidelberg approach the board of the IPP-Heidelberg-Mannheim for information. The board confronts the inquirers with its assessment that H. M.'s abstinence violations must have been known to the AKJP-Heidelberg for many years.
26. As soon as the accusations against H. M. became known, a small group of training candidates (approx. 4–7 people) formed at the AKJP-Heidelberg, who demanded that H. M. had to suspend his functions at the AKJP-Heidelberg as long as the suspicions remained. This demand meets with massive resistance within the institute, especially at management and staff level. Also from the side of the IPP-Heidelberg-Mannheim this group does not receive any reliable support.
27. At the end of February 1993 the case of "H. M." is discussed in detail at an extraordinary general meeting of the IPP-Heidelberg-Mannheim. Senior members of the AKJP-Heidelberg are also present.
28. At the beginning of March 1993, at a well-attended general meeting of the AKJP-Heidelberg, H. M. explained his perspective on the accusations against him – combined with the announcement that he would resign from his position at the AKJP-Heidelberg in about 2 years.
29. A lecturer at the AKJP-Heidelberg tells a colleague at an unspecified time (presumably in the wake of the discussions about H. M.'s resignation in 1993) that H. M. had already committed sexual assaults during his time in Berlin. This communication remains without consequences.

30. In March 1993, H. M. and his former patient, who is the mother of his daughter, marry. She is pregnant again at this time. On the occasion of the marriage some leading members (also board members) of AKJP-Heidelberg turn up as well-wishers (see case 21).
31. At the end of April 1993 H. M. is questioned by the Heidelberg Criminal Police. On the basis of information from the Youth Welfare Office, he is accused of sexually abusing minors (R. R. and E. M., who became pregnant by him). Due to H. M.'s clarification that the young women were already of age at the time of the sexual contacts, there is apparently no further investigation.
32. On the initiative of a former training candidate of the AKJP-Heidelberg, the case of "H. M." is discussed and critically explored in the Federal Board of the Association of Analytic Child and Adolescent Psychotherapy Institutes (VAKJP). The discussions lead to a letter to the members of the AKJP-Heidelberg demanding the immediate resignation of H. M., otherwise the continued existence of the institute would be endangered. This letter is signed by 21 members of the regional group Baden of the VAKJP (Vereinigung Analytischer Kinder- und Jugendlichen-Psychotherapeuten in Deutschland e. V.), who are advised in their initiative by the justiciary of the VAKJP – four of them are training candidates of the AKJP-Heidelberg. (Together with a few others, they form a small group at the AKJP-Heidelberg who are campaigning for the immediate dismissal of H. M. in the face of fierce resistance within the institute). The letter contains the remarkable passage: "Some of us have had knowledge of various abstinence violations and have remained silent, others have sensed the atmosphere of boundary violations, have overlooked them or have accepted them with ironic commentary".
33. At an extraordinary general meeting in May 1993, an important course was set: (1) H. M. asks for the termination of his contract at AKJP-Heidelberg already in August 1993. (2) A. A. is elected first chairwoman of the supporting association of AKJP-Heidelberg. (3) It is made clear that H. M. is explicitly not to be accused of any boundary violations against children. Corresponding rumours, which were mentioned in a letter of the board of the VAKJP, were groundless.
34. Subsequently, two essential lines of conflict regarding the evaluation of the "Causa H. M." intensify: The first runs between the two institutes IPP-Heidelberg-Mannheim and AKJP-Heidelberg; the second operates within AKJP-Heidelberg. While one side demands lasting massive consequences on H. M.'s professional practice and functions due to his serious abstinence violations, the other side tends to trivialize the proven abstinence violations and to doubt further – not officially known – boundary violations and assaults. This

side also takes the stance that there is nothing to be said against continuing to entrust H. M. with second sights and supervisions, whereby H. M.'s services to the Institute are also acknowledged.

35. In the following years, repeated attempts were made, especially by the board of the IPP-Heidelberg-Mannheim, to obtain a professional ban as well as a ban on expert activities for H. M. via the medical associations. Since the accusations made are not considered to be sufficiently well-founded due to the lack of statements by the victims, no consequences are drawn on the part of the chamber. Simultaneously, the IPP-Heidelberg-Mannheim repeatedly receives reports of serious misconduct by H. M.'s wife over the years. For reasons of personal dependency, however, she too does not provide any information that would justify a withdrawal of the license to practice medicine at the district government or a revocation of the expert's activity by the medical association.
36. In 1994 H. M. is asked by the board of the VAKJP – on the initiative of the chairman of the IPP-Heidelberg-Mannheim – to resign from his position as an expert. The board of experts decides against H. M.'s resignation. According to the VAKJP's legal advisor, the VAKJP's hands are tied as long as no clear evidence against H. M. is presented.
37. In a meeting of leading representatives of AKJP-Heidelberg and IPP-Heidelberg-Mannheim in March 1994, different knowledge about the transgressions of H. M. are made the cause of mutual reproaches. The representatives of AKJP-Heidelberg unanimously come to the conclusion that they do not want to take action against H. M.'s work as an expert. They justify this with social considerations in connection with the "young family" that H. M. had founded with the former patient.
38. An employee of the AKJP-Heidelberg informs other psychotherapists (former training candidates of the AKJP-Heidelberg) in the context of an intervision group that accusations of sexual abuse of "one or two" boys were also made against H. M.. At least one of the colleagues came to the conclusion that her patients who had been seen by H. M. for a second sight had not suffered any sexual boundary violations by him.
39. In 1994, during an open day, parents complain to a therapist at the educational counselling centre in Ebersbach (a former trainee at the AKJP-Heidelberg) about boundary violations committed against their children at the AKJP-Heidelberg. The therapist then decides that she no longer wants to have anything to do with the AKJP-Heidelberg. She informs a colleague, who in turn forwards the information about the boundary violation to the head of the institute (see case 27).

40. Also in 1994 (or early 1995) a child psychiatrist from Weinheim informs H. M. that parents had complained to her about him because he had masturbated their son. To the head of the institute of the AKJP-Heidelberg H. M. was indignant about these reproaches and explained his behaviour with usual medical examination practices (see case 28).

In 1995 H. M. opened a practice for psychosomatic medicine and psychotherapy in Seckach (Odenwald).

41. Probably in 1995, a mother informs the psychotherapist of her daughter, who is about 9 years old, that the girl was asked by H. M. in the course of a second sight whether her older sister's breast was already growing and whether her nipple was becoming firm. Neither the mother nor the psychotherapist (former training candidate at AKJP-Heidelberg) take action (see case 29).
42. In mid-1995, H. M. was largely deprived of the commissioning of evaluations of applications from the Rhine-Neckar district (this also included applications from Heidelberg) on the initiative of the head of the AKJP-Heidelberg institute. This is ultimately justified by the fact that the awarding of expert commissions in local proximity is generally unusual. It is unclear to what extent the Federal Association of Statutory Health Insurances (KBV), which was involved in this process, was explicitly informed about the background of the initiative.
43. In October 1996 Dr. M. P. informs the board of the AKJP-Heidelberg that there are preliminary proceedings against H. M. in Seckach. The accusation was that he had grabbed a 9-year-old boy between his legs (or in his trousers). It is to be assumed that the preliminary proceedings were discontinued (see case 30).
44. Around 1996, during an inpatient treatment at the psychosomatic clinic in Heidelberg, a patient reports to her therapist that she had been led by her outpatient psychotherapist H. M. into his bedroom. In the team meeting at the clinic, the therapist pleads that the patient should no longer be allowed to go to H. M. for psychotherapy. The clinic manager takes the opposite view (see case 31).
45. At an indeterminable point in time (presumably 1996/1997) a patient tells her psychotherapist that her now adolescent son had reported to her several years ago that H. M. had played with his penis during an examination. She had not taken this seriously at the time, although the boy had repeatedly spoken about it. The psychotherapist explained to his patient that her son had probably made accurate statements at the time (see case 20).

46. In April 1997, a letter signed by 49 members of the IPP-Heidelberg-Mannheim to the 1. chairman of the VAKJP points out that the continuing activity of H. M. as an expert of the Association of Statutory Health Insurances (KV) and as an expert advisor of the Psychotherapy Commission is regarded as "incompatible with our common professional ethos". In view of the abstinence violations mentioned in the letter, the addressee is requested to "bring about a long pending clarification". At the beginning of May 1997 the first chairman of the VAKJP asks the general meeting to vote on whether the letter should be read out. The meeting decides against it.
47. In June 1997 the mother of a boy contacted the head of the AKJP-Heidelberg Institute with the following information: In the course of an examination by H. M. in 1989 her then 7-year-old son had to take off his trousers, whereupon H. M. had looked at his penis. At that time, the mother had considered speaking to H. M. about this, as her son had subsequently appeared to be very distressed. However, she refrained from doing so (see case 15).
48. In July 1997 a staff member of the AKJP-Heidelberg reported in a team meeting about a colleague whose patient had told in therapy about the sexual assaults her son had suffered several years before in an examination situation by H. M. (see case 20). In the course of this team meeting, a total of five pieces of information brought to the Institute's attention in the years 1994–1997 about sexual boundary violations committed against boys by H. M. were collected and discussed (cases 15, 20, 27, 28, 30).
49. At an unspecified point in time, a staff member of the AKJP-Heidelberg informed a colleague that she had never left any of her therapy children alone with H. M. She had never introduced any child to H. M. without her being present. It is unclear to which period this communication refers. The employee otherwise expressed herself to her colleague very reservedly about the "case of H. M.", but gave the impression that she "knew quite a bit".
50. At an unspecified point in time, an 8-year-old girl reports to her mother after two sessions with H. M. that she does not want to go there anymore because it is "piggy". It remains unclear how the mother subsequently deals with this information (see case 26).
51. In the context of the AKJP-Heidelberg-internal group "Past – Present – Future", which took place in 2000, sexual boundary violations by H. M. against children were reported. In the course of this (and/or due to discussions in team meetings) two members of staff search through files (especially records of second sights) from the AKJP-Heidelberg for possible anomalies, as older colleagues had given corresponding indications of boundary violating examination practices. The results of this research were communicated back to

the group. In retrospect, one of the two staff members summarizes: "From the memories of the commission members (= Group "Past – Present – Future") as well as from the written anamnesis reports that H. M. himself had prepared, the impression arose in the commission that H. M. mixed his role as psychotherapeutic and medical diagnostician". It is further stated, among other things, that during the examinations by H. M., boys had to strip naked.

52. In the year 2000, an employee of the AKJP-Heidelberg receives information from a psychiatrist, to whom he reports about the events at the institute, that a relative of hers suffered sexual boundary violations by H. M. in the course of therapy in 1976 when she was a 15-year-old girl. It is not known when the girl disclosed to her relative and what consequences were drawn from this communication (see case 3).
53. In July 2000 an employee of the AKJP-Heidelberg confesses to the head of the institute that she had misjudged the events surrounding H. M. for a long time. She had to realize that she had been lied to. She knew a lot, but could not talk about it.
54. In April 2013, the mother of a now adult man, who had been examined by H. M. as a boy in 1989, contacted both the AKJP-Heidelberg and the VAKJP in order to obtain information about the events of that time. In this context, either the mother or the victim filed a criminal complaint against H. M., but the investigations were discontinued (see case 19).
55. Due to a complaint filed by his daughter with the North Baden District Medical Association, H. M.'s medical license is revoked with effect from 01.01.2014. The accusations refer to paedosexual tendencies and corresponding photo and video material. H. M. initially denies these facts, but then returns his licence to practise medicine. There are no indications that the allegations made have led to criminal investigations. H. M. is then prohibited from all medical activities, including the writing of expert opinions. It subsequently became clear that H. M. did not adhere to these conditions and continued to write expert opinions.
56. Around 2015, a psychotherapist tells her supervisor about "perverted video recordings" that her patient's father makes of her daughter (i.e. his grandchild). The supervisor verifies that the grandfather is H. M.. Since the patient does not release her therapist from confidentiality, the case cannot be uncovered or reported. However, it could be that the patient's decision to report her father, realized a year later, came about because of the support of her therapist.
57. In June 2016, one of H. M. s daughters filed criminal charges against her father for sexually abusing her daughter, who was 4 years old at the time (see Case 32).

58. Around the end of 2016/2017 there are considerations at AKJP-Heidelberg to reach persons who were in treatment with H. M. (or for second sight) via a public call. However, this initiative will not be pursued further.
59. In March 2017, the defendant H. M. is proven to have committed sexual abuse against his granddaughter in 11 cases. He is sentenced to a suspended sentence of 18 months. Despite corresponding efforts, in particular by the ethics officer of AKJP-Heidelberg, the boundary violations of H. M. in the context of his professional activity at AKJP-Heidelberg are not the subject of the trial. On the fringes of the trial, there are several reports of H. M.'s earlier boundary violations, which are voiced in the circle of former and current members of the institute.
60. Through the publication of an article in the weekly newspaper "Die ZEIT" (published on 16.08.2018), which was researched in the course of the court case against H. M., the extent of H. M.'s deeds (against teaching analysts, young female patients and children) becomes known to a larger public, at least to some extent.

The potential for disclosure listed here should first be seen from the point of view of prevention. The urgent question arises as to whether consistent disclosure of boundary violations and assaults at earlier points in time would have led to the prevention of a large number of further acts, some of which were associated with serious harm to girls, boys and women. This question not least constitutes the evaluation framework within which the situations described here are to be located. The question of what prevented sustained disclosures over such long periods of time will be the subject of detailed discussions below. At this point, only a few descriptive observations may be made: The overall picture is one of many potential strands of disclosure leading unconnectedly into the void. Many people suspect something, many express or receive concrete indications of deeds, that in their isolated evaluation obviously causes great difficulties. One should not fall prey to the belief that the 60 potentials for disclosure presented here completely depict the discursive events surrounding H. M.'s boundary violations. Rather, the assumption emerges that this list has an exemplary character for qualitative aspects of corresponding communications, but does not provide any information about the extent of what was perceived, thought, implied, spoken and heard within professional and private sub-publics.

Distinct social segments can be sketched here, within which the language of disclosure repeatedly came to a standstill over a long period of time:

- In the first segment there are parents who took note of their sons' and daughters' reports about "strange examination methods" of the doctor H. M. and in many cases remained alone with it.
- The second segment is populated by psychotherapists who receive a variety of information about their colleague's transgressions in the treatment setting and see themselves condemned in the secrecy of the psychoanalytic method to helplessly circle around such information. Thus, one interviewee reports how she/he told her/his teaching analyst about suspicions against H.M.:

> I mean, that's the shit, I'm going to say now (laughs), you can't say to the analyst in such a case in your own analysis, you have to say something now. I can say, you have to say something now – not you, but you have to say something now – but he might not say anything.

- The respective institute publics at IPP-Heidelberg-Mannheim and at AKJP-Heidelberg form a further segment. For a long time, this segment is characterized by a discourse that has to remain vague in order to keep the noise of suspicion alive without revealing any actual need for action.
- The fourth segment is made up of external bodies: Youth Welfare Office, police, umbrella organizations, health insurance companies. One can by no means say that the AKJP-Heidelberg constituted a hermetic complex from which no hints about H. M.'s deeds would have leaked out. On the contrary, external instances were – at least from 1992 onwards – included in the discourse about H. M. in many different ways. But also in this segment strands are formed which come to nothing: Criminal charges are filed, the Youth Welfare Office apparently sees considerable indications of danger, health insurance companies and umbrella organizations are obviously supplied with a great deal of information which justifies the need for action in dealing with H. M., but which is not taken up.
- The fifth segment is constituted by the operational management level of the institutes AKJP-Heidelberg and IPP-Heidelberg-Mannheim as well as by the boards of the supporting associations. This segment, too, does not seem to be sufficiently connected with the other social structures in which indications of dangers from H. M. are virulent.
- The last segment can be described as the "Heidelberg psychotherapy scene", which can be institutionally located in various clinics and in the private practices of therapists. Naturally, there are relevant overlaps with the institutes AKJP-Heidelberg and IPP-Heidelberg-Mannheim. But these overlaps do not

seem to contribute, at least for a long time, to bringing together circulating strands of information in the sense of a coordinated disclosure strategy.

From these observations the finding can be derived that there are manifold potentials for uncovering that fall flat. In fact, until the end of 1992, there was no recognizable attempt to seriously and critically discuss, let alone put an end to, the frequently disclosed transgressions, assaults, abstinence violations, and the abuse of power perpetrated by sexual means. The indications which led to H. M.'s removal as head of the institute in 1993 can at best be described as fragmentary in view of the multitude and massiveness of the acts committed by him up to that time. Nevertheless, they justified an at least partially successful uncovering action. Later attempts to critically discuss and scandalize were also based on circumstantial evidence, which became identifiable on the basis of comparatively thin and poorly contoured strands of information. Thus, any attempt at disclosure had to be accompanied by weighty doubts, since the overall picture did not open up. The isolation of the social and institutional segments described above was only lifted in a few places, so that no comprehensive disclosure process could develop. As an example for that, see those cases mentioned here in which psychotherapists confided in colleagues with the information that they had been told a long time ago by patients that they in turn had learned a long time ago from their children that they had experienced sexual assaults by H. M. in the examination or treatment situation. But not every communication requires decades to penetrate the thick walls of shame and fear. We also learn that H. M. discloses the birth of a boy at the Institute, the result of his relationship with a young female patient whose therapy had just ended. Brazen revelations constitute just as petered out strands of disclosure as the decades-long delays in communication by affected children, their parents, and their treating psychotherapists.

The events of omission outlined here take their form through isolated strands of information that circulate at different time levels in social segments that are separated from one another. How these formations, which prevented a sustained exposure of H. M.'s deeds, developed, will be analyzed below.

4.4 Attempts of Inquiry

As described above, in the present context, for reasons of clarity, a separation is made between disclosure and inquiry on a purely descriptive level. In fact, however, it can be seen that attempts of inquiry were often associated with elements of disclosure, and disclosure events in turn raised the awareness of individuals of the need for systematic inquiry.

1. In September 1993, M. P. stated in a letter to G. C., the then chairman of the IPP-Heidelberg-Mannheim, that a course was offered at the AKJP-Heidelberg "to work through the problem" and that a discussion group had been formed which would be open to all those involved.
2. In the middle of December 1993 there is "a short review" of the events which led to the resignation of H. M. at a general meeting of the AKJP-Heidelberg. The wish is expressed that at least one member of the AKJP-Heidelberg board should talk to the member of the board of the IPP-Heidelberg-Mannheim, who acts as a direct contact person for the women who were affected. This is connected with the hope of gaining clarity about the accusations against H. M..
3. In March 1994 the above-mentioned discussion between leading representatives of the two institutes AKJP-Heidelberg and IPP-Heidelberg-Mannheim took place. In the minutes it is stated that an unpleasant but necessary work had been done by discussing the "facts".
4. In the spring of 1994, the IPP-Heidelberg-Mannheim is planning a workshop on the topic of "Boundary Violations in Psychotherapy".
5. In the course of 1994 there are two little-attended meetings at AKJP-Heidelberg, which are not explicitly declared as general meetings. In one of these meetings the possibility of an inquiry in the form of group supervision is discussed. This idea is also pushed by a board member of the VAKJP. In January 1995, a participant of these meetings (former training candidate at the AKJP-Heidelberg) proposes in a letter to the director of the institute the initiation of group supervision in the sense mentioned.
6. In July 1996, at a general meeting of the AKJP-Heidelberg, the demand for an external supervision in order to come to terms with the events at the Institute was raised again. The director of the institute as well as the chairwoman of the board point out that this attempt had already been made once, but that hardly anyone had signed the list posted in the seminar room.
7. In 1997 the annual conference of the VAKJP is held in Heidelberg under the deliberately chosen theme "Traumatized Children and Adolescents – Theory and Treatment". The regional group Baden regards this as a contribution to working through the events surrounding H. M..
8. At the end of April 1998, in a conversation between the head of the institute and several members of staff, the question of an inquiry of that part of the history of the AKJP-Heidelberg which concerns the case of H. M. is raised. Subsequently, two members of staff submitted a motion for the general meeting of the AKJP-

Heidelberg in June 1998, in which they raised the problem that the discussions about H. M. at the AKJP-Heidelberg had been silent for 3 years, that in the meantime at least three cases had become known in which H. M. had committed sexual assaults against boys, and that H. M. continued to work as an expert witness for the KV and as an expert advisor to the Psychotherapy Commission and ran a psychotherapy practice for adults, children and adolescents in Seckach. As the general meeting did not seem to them to be the appropriate body, two members of staff proposed the establishment of an ethics committee to deal with the incidents.

9. In June 1999, these two employees of the AKJP-Heidelberg request the prompt convening of an extraordinary general meeting in order to decide on the exclusion of H. M. from the supporting association of the AKJP-Heidelberg. In the context of the ordinary general meeting, two board members of AKJP-Heidelberg announce that they would like to offer a group for all those members who would like an inquiry of the incidents surrounding H. M..

In August 1999 H. M. terminates his membership in the supporting association of AKJP-Heidelberg.

10. Meetings of the AKJP-Heidelberg-internal group "Past – Present – Future" will be held in 2000 (dates: 12.1.; 22.02.; 05.04.; 17.05.; 12.07.; 11.10.; 13.12.). This group is facilitated by board member M.K.. Many former and current members of AKJP-Heidelberg participate in the group. A protocol of the discussions is omitted. In a letter of December 2000 the members of the AKJP-Heidelberg are informed about the course of the group: "After clarification and inquiry processes concerning the past of the Institute (1st–4th evening), the discussion group devoted itself in the 2nd part of its work (5th–7th round) to questions of the members concerning the scientific location, the external effect and the identity of the Institute". A summary of the last meeting shows that the Causa H. M. was not discussed at this meeting.
11. Presumably in connection with the group "Past – Present – Future" the above mentioned search of files of the AKJP-Heidelberg by two employees of the institute takes place. It is not recognizable that the information generated by this stimulates further inquiry efforts.
12. In November 2002 the AKJP-Heidelberg organizes a conference on the occasion of its 50th anniversary with the title "Successfully Growing Up Today". Especially in the context of a panel discussion the case of "H. M." becomes the subject of partly emotional discussions.

13. In 2004, the Director of the Institute will offer a seminar for AKJP-Heidelberg training candidates, which deals with the history of the institute and also explicitly with the "Causa H. M.".
14. In April 2010, at the request of one of the two, a member of staff is elected as ethics officer of AKJP-Heidelberg at a general meeting.
15. In July 2013, a lecture and discussion event at IPP-Heidelberg-Mannheim (together with the Heidelberg institutes HIT and HIP) will discuss "problematic treatment-related constellations that lead to complaints or boundary violations" with the DGPT's trust analyst Giulietta Tibone.
16. In November 2016, the director of the institute and the ethics officer offered a seminar for AKJP-Heidelberg trainees about the boundary violations committed by H. M. and the findings and consequences to be drawn from them. In the run-up to this event, the head of the IPP Institute Heidelberg-Mannheim had expressed concern that J. S. and A. A. were appropriating the history of the AKJP Institute Heidelberg in a way that contributed to the denial of H. M.'s deeds.
17. In July 2017, H. M.'s wife offers the head of the AKJP-Heidelberg Institute diary records of H. M. in which boundary violations are described. The head of the institute discusses this offer with the ethics officer. At an earlier point in time, which cannot be determined, H. M.'s wife had given a former version of H. M.'s diary to an executive of the IPP-Heidelberg-Mannheim. At a later point in time, she passed the diary on to her successor as ethics officer of the DGPT. The numerous pieces of information about sexual boundary violations contained therein were not used against H. M..
18. From the seminar offered at the end of 2016, a group of former and current members of the Institute is constituted at AKJP-Heidelberg, which takes on the task of inquirying the case of H. M..
19. Related to the court case against H. M. for sexual abuse of his granddaughter (March 2017), the lawyer of H. M.'s wife contacts a journalist from the weekly newspaper "Die ZEIT" who is researching this matter. The journalist contacted the then ethics officer of the AKJP-Heidelberg. Die "ZEIT" researched extensively in H. M.'s institutional environment about his boundary violations and assaults committed there. Among other things, the role of the AKJP Institute Heidelberg and various protagonists of the Heidelberg psychotherapy scene are discussed. Within these contexts, a further dynamization of the conflict occurred after the publication of the article on August 16, 2018.
20. At the IPP Heidelberg-Mannheim (training institute of the DPG in Heidelberg), after the court case, considerations are made to deal intensively with the "Causa H. M.", since many members had done their training at the IPP-

Heidelberg-Mannheim. However, no concrete initiatives were taken in this regard. All those involved were members of the DGP.

21. The ethics officer of the AKJP Heidelberg filed a criminal complaint against H. M. in 2017 because he continued to work as an expert witness. Investigations were started in this matter, but H. M. died before proceedings were opened.
22. On the initiative of the AKJP-Heidelberg inquiry group, a decision was taken at a general meeting of the AKJP-Heidelberg at the end of 2018 to commission the Institute for Practice Research and Project Consulting Munich (IPP Munich) with the systematic inquiry of the "Causa H. M.". This was done against the resistance of a group of members, especially from J. S.'s environment, who expressed concerns about the associated financial burdens and the reputation of the institute in the public.
23. IPP Munich starts the scientific inquiry of the "Causa H. M." in February 2019.

In March 2019, H. M. passes away at the age of 86.

On a descriptive level, it should first be noted that the number of inquiry initiatives in the aftermath of the revelations in 1993 is enormous. On the surface, one could say that since then, more than 20 attempts have been made from various sides to take the necessary step of a conscious institutional reflection on the incidents surrounding H. M.. This is not surprising in view of the fact that we are moving in a professional environment whose central methodology consists in becoming aware of past events. Against this background, therefore, the insight that there is a need for inquiry was formulated in various places at an early stage. Based on this observation, however, a picture is forming that is not dissimilar to the one described above related to disclosure potentials: Initiatives placed in various systems that fall flat in ways that are initially difficult to comprehend. Examples of this are suggestions in relation to group supervision in the 1990s and the establishment of an ethics committee at AKJP-Heidelberg, which did not happen until 2010. A series of events was held in which the "Causa H. M." was discussed, which was apparently associated with short-term but unsystematic processes of awareness and also disclosure among individuals in the environment of the institutes AKJP-Heidelberg and IPP-Heidelberg-Mannheim. The IPP-Heidelberg-Mannheim claims to have regularly made boundary violations and abstinence violations in the psychoanalytic setting the subject of well-attended events. On the basis of the data available to us, this cannot be proven beyond doubt, but on the other hand it cannot be falsified either. The group "Past – Present – Future" at AKJP-Heidelberg in 2000 can be interpreted as an "index event" for institutional inquiry. On the level of institutional symptomatology, however, several phenomena can be identified which make it clear that the variously associated claim with this group to investigate has failed comprehensively:

1. Within the group, sexual boundary violations by H. M. against children and adolescents were discussed. The fact that H. M. was running a psychotherapeutic practice for children, adolescents and adults at this time did not trigger any impulses for action in the direction of child protection on the part of the group.
2. In retrospect, leading members of the group "forgot" that H. M.'s sexual boundary violations against children and adolescents had even been discussed there. This emerges beyond doubt from our interviews.
3. In the last session of the group, the "case of H. M." was no longer discussed at all. The movement in terms of content increasingly went in a methodological-professional direction, so that the impression arises that the mode of keeping silent about H. M.'s boundary violations "tacitly" gained more and more space.
4. Already two years later, at an event on the occasion of the 50th anniversary of the AKJP-Heidelberg, the massively different emotional and ethical interpretations of the "H. M. case" became visible to the public. At the latest, these disputes should have led to a conscious retrospective questioning of the group's meaningfulness and effectiveness.
5. Also in the following years, a still existing conflict dynamic, which was ignited by the "Causa H. M.", manifested itself again and again.

Of particular interest is the intensification of the long dormant process of working through the past more than 20 years after the disclosures that took place in 1993. First of all, it should be noted that the intensity of the associated conflicts and the dynamics between impulses for action and resistance indicate quite clearly that all the attempts at an institutional inquiry initiated up to that point did not fulfil the expectations associated with them. The court case against H. M. and the publication of the "ZEIT" article can be claimed as further "index events" which made the need of an institutional self-reflection – even about 25 years after H. M. left the institutes IPP-Heidelberg-Mannheim and AKJP-Heidelberg – recognizable.

5 Conceptual Framework for the Classification of Events

In this section, some concepts are discussed that contribute to an orientation with regard to the classification of the sexual boundary violations and sexual relations initiated by H. M. Since we are dealing with a plethora of case constellations related to H. M., a conceptual classification is needed in order to theoretically grasp the problem discussed here and thus contribute to an improved understanding of the processes at the psychoanalytic institutes AKJP-Heidelberg and IPP-Heidelberg-Mannheim.

5.1 Normality

The concept of normality is as intuitive as it is demanding. Asserted normality forms a frame of reference to which the evaluation of perceptions and observations is often oriented. This by no means implies that the "normal" is regularly equated with the "positive", but normality nonetheless establishes a certain cultural convention to which a relevant argumentative power is attributed. For the context discussed here, it is important to refer back to notions of normality in relation to sexuality and sexual violence (cf. Araji, 1997; Schuhrke, 2002). The distinction between different dimensions of normality proves to be meaningful insofar as their non-consideration leads to misunderstandings and blockades to action in relation to suspicions or cases of sexual violence. One interview partner expresses this as follows:

P. Caspari et al., *At some point there has to be peace and quiet!*,
https://doi.org/10.1007/978-3-658-39785-2_5

> And now it's also quite simple, I just have more experience. My horizons have already broadened considerably from back then, so I find this form of naivety impressive (laughs) when I look back at all the things I didn't see.

In the present context, a distinction is made between four different dimensions of normality in order to discursively frame the different case constellations at issue (cf. Mosser, 2012): (1) morally grounded normality, (2) penologically grounded normality, (3) health-related normality, (4) statistical normality.

5.1.1 Morally Based Normality

This dimension describes the area that we "intuitively" associate with normality. Normal is "what is proper", whereby such judgments are aimed at a subjective moral sense that is biographically and socially formed. This sense is activated, for example, when there is cause for moral outrage. Events are then judged as "abnormal", "deviant" or "perverse". In connection with H. M.'s acts, a kind of reflexive marginalization of the moral argument is generally observable: the sexual assaults against children and adolescents are for a long time either completely dismissed or relegated to the realm of medically justified action. On the other hand, H. M.'s relationships with training candidates and teaching analysands, which were already known at an early stage, release moral feelings which – as it often appears in the interviews – have to be actively "whistled back": These are matters between adults. That the women with whom H. M. engages in sexual relations are married cannot be a cause for moral outrage. Nor can the fact that he may be having multiple relationships at the same time. It is as if the largescale retraction of the moral argument simultaneously swept all that is problematic about these relationships even beyond the moral argument into an all-encompassing argumentative abyss in which it is no longer possible to talk at all about what is going on before the eyes of an extensive institutional public. The "Zeitgeist" contributed its share to the fact that anyone who was morally outraged by the institute director, who was obviously very interested in women, could end up on the social sidelines. What is interesting here is two things: a comprehensive tabooing of moral feeling (as if one were arguing unprofessionally when one argues morally) and an abrupt flare-up of the moral argument the moment one allows the realization that H. M.'s "touching" of children can no longer be accommodated in categories of "normal" medical practice. In most cases, however, this initially leads to a defensive reaction: "I didn't know that he did anything with children, too!" These defensive reactions are accompanied by the speculative assumption that moral outrage and correspondingly consistent action would have been activated if only one had known about it (cf. Mitscherlich & Mitscherlich, 2007). Around the "ZEIT" article an astonished extended institute public is grouped, which cannot grasp that H. M. has also committed offences against children. At this point there is now the permission for moral indignation, which one denied oneself in view of what was allowed to be known in all the decades before. This denial weighs most heavily in view of the relationship between H. M. and his (ex-)patient E. M. The fact that an old man, especially a psychotherapeutically active doctor and respected institute director, has a love affair with a woman almost 40 years younger, pushes back the moral sentiment at the moment when it prepares to evoke indignation. One is "enlightened" enough not to take offence at something that one's own parents' generation, which one is proud to have overcome, would probably still have been terribly upset about. Again, there is the risk of a generalized defense of moral judgment: If what would qualify as "indecent" about it in a way that cannot be described in detail is excluded from the moral judgment, then the power relationship between the old doctor and the young woman, which is obviously out of joint and considering that the woman was socialized in the youth welfare system, does not need to be problematized any further either. Just how strong the effect of the averted moral judgement is becomes apparent at the moment when the marriage between the two is announced. As strong as the irritation at this grotesque move was, it is now clear that the moral argument has remained quite powerful. In fact, a kind of "reassurance" about the fact that H. M. subsequently "legitimized" his relationship with his (ex-)patient by marrying her sets in at influential positions of AKJP-Heidelberg. The fact that he is "obviously serious" about the relationship with the young woman is a judgement that appeals solely to those moral sentiments that previously had to be warded off.

5.1.2 Criminal Normality

The criminal law does not explicitly define normality, but it does provide important orientations regarding the assessment of whether something is normal or not. That these orientations are changeable is shown by a superficial look at the history of sexual criminal law, in which, for example, the assessment of homosexual acts, the sanctioning of sexual violence in the context of marriage or sexual violence against men have been subject to fundamental changes within a time frame not very long ago (Rohne & Wirths, 2018). Criminal law-based norm-setting was certainly significant in relation to H.M.'s acts at various points and was also repeatedly introduced into the discussion: the sexual abuse of children, which H. M. could ultimately be proven to have committed through his crime against his granddaughter, could have been invoked as a criminal offence at any time. As far as is known, corresponding investigations were therefore also initiated at least twice, which were, however, prematurely discontinued. This initially points to a very powerful discrepancy between criminal law norms and criminal law practice (cf. Jehle, 2012). However, this does not change the fact that all of H. M. 's sexual acts against minors were in principle punishable. The "insignificance" or the "medical-therapeutic justifiability" turn out to be hair-raising argumentative chimeras in view of what is known by now. With respect to his relationships with adult women (even with some of them young women), criminal law-based standard-setting proves more ambiguous. The question of whether an institute director may engage in sexual relations with female training candidates or even female teaching analysts and patients escaped any criminal law assessment until 1998 (cf. Schleu et al., 2018). Starting points for investigations could only have arisen in the case of demonstrably violent sexual acts, i.e. sexual coercion or rape.

5.1.3 Health-Related Normality

For the cases to be examined here, health norms may play the greatest role. What qualifies as "normal" in the sexual sphere may be based on whether there is a risk of harm to the health of a person involved. For sexual acts between adults and minors, this is regularly the case and requires no further discussion (see Mosser, 2018). In the analysis of the events surrounding H. M., it is noteworthy that the "health argument" was only marginally introduced into the discussion with regard to the young women who were impregnated by him. At least in relation to E. M. this represents an astonishing omission, since she was a psychotherapeutic patient who was obviously struggling with health problems. When such a young woman becomes involved in a sexual relationship by her psychotherapist, there is actually acute cause for concern – and not only among the relevant professional public – about her mental health.[1] (Becker-Fischer & Fischer, 1996) It is interesting to note here that in the controversy surrounding the case, recourse was made more to issues of criminal law or professional ethics and less to the potential for harm inherent in this relationship, which was obvious to all. The health argument in particular was pushed back in the psychotherapeutic discourse arena, while much more

[1]The same applies to the mother of H. M.'s son, born in 1980. She too was a former patient, very young and also cared for by the youth welfare service. Surprisingly, this relationship did not lead to any consequences, not even to any inquiries, neither in the institute nor in the extended public of the institute.

attention was paid to pragmatic questions of institutional handling. As if there were no further – ethically justified – mandate for action at the moment when the damage to health through marriage is "privatized". In comparison, the importance of the health argument was clearly emphasized in the context of the women who had been sexually exploited by H. M. in the context of training relationships and teaching analyses. The fact that, according to the information provided by the director of the IPP-Heidelberg-Mannheim whom they had taken into their confidence, the women concerned had suffered severely from the effects of their relationships with H. M., was very clearly brought into the discussion by those who called for consequences for H. M. In this way, an attempt was made to raise awareness of the fact that these were not simply relationships between adults. This also invalidated H. M.'s account that the relationships had only begun after the completion of the teaching analyses. Here, at the latest, it becomes clear that health normality can by no means always be brought into agreement with moral normality, but that they are independent dimensions which must be reflected upon separately in the evaluation of social phenomena, in particular also in the evaluation of abstinence violations in the context of psychotherapies.[2] The fact that abstinence violations damage the health of patients by contaminating the therapy is also expressed in the following assessment by a representative of the adult institute:

> There have been countless seminars on this, and I think that's right. And not because it's about any morals, but because the transference doesn't work, it gets very disturbed, when someone as an analyst tells about his life out of his own need, then the transference is so disturbed, so that was the motive, not a moral motive.

However, in the different treatment of the various abstinence violations, a moral differentiation of the health aspect among the contemporary witnesses is noticeable. Despite their known need for treatment, the young female patients were not in the focus when it came to the health-damaging consequences of the boundary violations by H. M. This argument was almost exclusively used in connection with the (soon to be) own guild training candidates or teaching analysands.

---

[2] See, however, Krutzenbichler's (1998) remark with reference to the serious damage to health caused by sexual transgressions in psychotherapy, according to which "it is not the actually occurring consequences, but the conscious acceptance of these possible consequences for the sake of satisfying a personal need (…) that (determines) such action as profoundly unethical" (p. 321).

5.1.4 Statistical Normality

This dimension refers to an argument that what is normal is what is common. What at first seems hardly contestable raises complicated questions at second glance. For example, the growing evidence over the past decades that sexual violence by clergy was common (Dreßing et al., 2018) would tend not to suggest that it was a normal occurrence (as moral, penal, and health-related notions of normality suggest discrepant judgments). In the course of our interviews, we sometimes heard it suggested that there are "many" instances of psychotherapists sexually exploiting female patients or initiating sexual relationships with teaching analysts or training candidates.[3] The reference to the sheer frequency of the occurrence of such constellations seems optionally to serve two argumentative functions: Either as an indication of the seriousness of the problem and the risks associated with the psychotherapeutic setting, or as a "defusing" of the specific case of H. M.: Implicitly, it is suggested here that there is no need for the special fuss, since a more pragmatic way of dealing with similar cases has finally been found elsewhere. To put it bluntly, this means: In a sense, because such cases are not rare, they are "normal" (cf. Bittner, 1998). Such assertions of normality also provided a framework for evaluation in the 1970s and 1980s, for example, when the lecturer K. H. had a sexual relationship with a female trainee and it was also heard from other institutes that relationships between lecturers and trainees were not unusual. Possibly one was involved in such relationship constellations oneself, possibly one was in love with one's analysand as a teaching analyst, possibly the construction of normality in relation to H. M.'s behaviour had an effective function of protecting one's own self. The subsequent horror at the fact that H. M. had also committed sexual acts against children leaves one's own notions of normality, according to which sexual relations can sometimes occur in the life of an institute, untouched. Such notions of frequency can corrupt moral or health-related orientations to normality by statistically legitimizing what is actually rejected, so to speak (even if it is only in the form of presumed dark figures).

It becomes clear that both internal and discursively negotiated notions of normality played an important role in dealing with the "Causa H. M.". This is astonishing insofar as the image that is formed in retrospective observation of this case cannot be reconciled with any notions of normality that would have a chance of social agreement. It can be assumed that the conscious or unconscious fading out of certain dimensions of normality made a significant contribution both to the

[3] See Hirsch (2012), "It is fair to say that today every therapist knows of one or more cases of massive narcissistic and sexual abuse from their immediate or wider environment" (p. 35).

resistance to disclosure in relation to H. M.'s actions and to institutional blockades to action in the wake of individual acts and relationship constellations becoming known (cf. Burka et al., 2019; Sandler & Godley, 2004).

5.2 Professional Ethics: Organizational Ethics

In retrospect of the different periods in which H. M. worked at the AKJP-Heidelberg and at the IPP-Heidelberg-Mannheim and in which the institutes had to deal with his case, changes in discursive references are noticeable. First of all it has to be stated that until 1993 there was obviously no reliable possibility of orientation at the AKJP-Heidelberg, which would have made it possible to evaluate H. M.'s behaviour, which had become more or less known.

According to the information of an expert whom we interviewed in the context of our research on the development of the corresponding discourse, the handling of sexualized interactions within psychotherapies was intensively discussed in the psychotherapy associations in the 1990s at the latest:

> Well, we discussed that. 94 I had already had many discussions, so I would have known that it was definitely wrong (…). And for the [psychoanalysts, author's note] dependence was the central concept. So that's why I say they actually had a more intensive ethical discussion.

This deficit of information, judgement and action at the AKJP-Institute Heidelberg can be summarized in terms of professional ethics and organizational ethics. As a central criterion for the professional ethical self-positioning of all those who worked at the IPP-Heidelberg-Mannheim and at the AKJP-Heidelberg (both as teachers and learners), the concept of abstinence should be mentioned, to which more detailed explanations will be devoted below. Professional ethics refers to a positively formulated set of values that fundamentally constitute the self-understanding of a particular profession (cf. Hutterer-Krisch, 2007; Schleu & Habenicht, 2014). In this context, the question often arises as to the extent to which such ethical standards remain rather implicit or are repeatedly updated in professional action and thus provide grounds for corresponding social validation. In this regard, Krutzenbichler's, 1998 observation that there is no code of psychoanalytic ethics "and certainly no universally accepted one" (p. 320) is noteworthy. One could say that psychoanalytic treatment is virtually predestined for the explication of professional ethical problems due to the multitude of questions that cluster around the interpretation of the abstinence rule.[4] (Tibone & Schmieder-Dembek, 2015) In our interviews, we gained the impression that the psychotherapeutic setting with children seems to be associated with rather implicit professional ethical self-locations and rarely releases conscious self-inquiries as in the following example:

> So I have another children's therapy room and I have my place behind the table (laughs), then the table in front of it and then the child there. And in between is the playhouse. But then they come now and then – then they try to come to me like that, so you have to position yourself very clearly. And I think you have to communicate that very clearly in the supervision sessions, what you can and can't do.

Since sexual boundary violations against girls or boys in psychotherapeutic treatment are obviously beyond the imagination of many psychotherapists, orientations in this regard initially appear uncomplicated. The answer to the question of whether a crying child may be taken in one's arms or whether one can pat a young person on the shoulder with encouragement is possibly delegated to the realm of personal intuition. Many things seem "clear" because personal feelings seem to provide orientation.

It is important to understand that such self-locations actually refer to elementary questions of professional ethics that require explicit discourse (cf. VAKJP, 2001). This becomes clear at the latest when one thinks of the doctor and psychotherapist H. M., who demands that children strip naked. It seems almost hair-raising that within the public of the institute the question was apparently never seriously raised as to what the head of the institute actually does in the course of hundreds or thousands of second sights. Since the second sight records left no doubt that H. M. saw the penises of boys, these should have given cause for professional ethical self-questioning of his colleagues and training candidates. Is H. M. allowed to do this "as a doctor"? Can it be part of psychotherapeutic diagnostics to question children about their masturbation experiences? How do you talk to adolescent patients about their sexuality? Can it be part of the psychoanalytic treatment technique to induce feelings of shame in underage patients? And if so, to what extent? If such questions were ever asked, they were delegated to the exclusive or clandestine space of supervision. Regardless of the extent to which the orientations elaborated there were helpful, the instrument of supervision appears, at least in retrospect, as

[4] Körner (1998a) assigns the abstinence rule the indispensable function of an element within a psychoanalytic triad: "The rules prohibit the use of the other, they are – especially as a framework of the situation – the "third", which is withdrawn from the arbitrariness of the two participants" (p. 341).

a symptom of the fragmentation of the professional ethical discourse. Nothing happened there that would have given rise to a critical questioning of the psychotherapeutic actions of the director of the institute. Other questions could have been asked: "Is it compatible with the ethical principles of our profession to initiate sexual relations with (young) patients after the end of psychotherapy?" "How much time must pass after the end of therapy before one is allowed to do so?" "How big can the age difference between the participants be?" "Are sexual relationships between teaching analysts and teaching analysands professionally acceptable?" (cf. Schleu et al., 2018). One can answer such questions intuitively by drawing on personal feelings. In this context, one of the experts we interviewed argues for an anticipatory belief in the infallibility of psychotherapists – at least in earlier times:

> I think that in the 80s the image was still actually that we were doing a good job and actually assuming that we were good people. Who else does a job like that? And so a professional self-image only slowly developed about what to do, boundaries of what to do.

If, however, the questions raised above are not discussed on the basis of professional ethics, but are assessed "emotionally", then figures of discourse emerge in an institutional public sphere that maraud around unconnectedly, such as those of the "one-time slip", of the "head of the institute who fascinates the women" and of the "doctor who is also allowed to touch the children during the examination".

At this point, the importance of organizational ethical issues becomes visible. This relates to the culture of a respective organization and thus to "shared assumptions, values, beliefs and norms on the basis of which appropriate and inappropriate behaviour is distinguished" (Christmann & Wazlawik, 2019, p. 237). This points to the need for a transfer of professional ethical discourses into the respective organizational contexts in which they find practical application, so to speak. What is meant by this is a "continuous self-reflective examination of one's own cultures, structures, dynamics, rules and attitudes as a long-term organizational and quality development process" (ibid. p. 239). Organizational ethics initially includes an "object-related dimension, on which both the topics to be ethically negotiated are marked and the structural elements available in an organization are named" (p. 242). In addition, there is a need for a decidedly process-oriented component associated with the task of "making ethical issues and processes of negotiation consistently accessible through 'organized spaces, rules, contexts, and rituals of shared discussion'" (ibid. p. 242). These remarks point to the extent of failures that characterized AKJP-Heidelberg over a long period of time. In this context, the critical retrospective is not to be invalidated by the argument that there were no established discourses on organizational ethics in the 1970s/1980s; rather, it is necessary to recall what is meant by "organizational ethics" and what undoubtedly should have been part of the repertoire of every psychotherapeutic training institute even back then. The question of institutional self-understanding and institutional self-location cannot be exhausted in the discussion about the preferred psychoanalytic method of treatment. Precisely because it is a type of organization in which high standards of professional ethics are valid and in which interpersonal relationships function as the central point of reference for one's professional actions, what is called "organizational ethics" must be reflected upon in the sense described above: "How do we treat each other here?" "What are the rules here?", "What are our attitudes?". Possibly, however, it is not only true for AKJP-Heidelberg that the transformation of formally established professional ethical standards (e.g. of the DGPT or the VAKJP) into an organizational ethics of the respective institutes is not sufficiently developed.

The consistent avoidance of a reliable discourse on organizational ethics at AKJP-Heidelberg seems symptomatic in retrospect. Far from speaking here of a deliberate "perpetrator strategy", it nevertheless becomes clear that the absence of a declared organizational ethic contributed to the fact that the actions of all those involved were essentially left to their own discretion. In the absence of an appropriate frame of reference, a system of ethical isolation emerged within which many things became possible: Dancing closely with the institute director at the institute party, dancing bare-breasted on the table, observing amorous initiations, hanging up photos of trips with (former) training candidates and/or teaching analysts in the institute rooms, revealing "spicy stuff" from the institute director's private life as a secretary at the institute, etc.... And if one's training is recognized and one receives a license to practice with the friendly assistance of the director of the institute, even if not all the requirements are met, then one's willingness to come to terms with the "peculiarities" of the institute (and its director) increases. Some took offence at these peculiarities, some wondered, some were "not so closely connected with the institute", but nobody seemed to demand a systematic discourse about the professional laws according to which that institute, in which one worked and/or completed one's psychotherapeutic training, actually functioned. The fact that the director of the institute himself had no interest in such a discussion is not worth explaining further, given the fact that this "organizational culture" gave him unrestricted power, sexual contacts, a high reputation and financial advantages. Obviously, however, other people who worked at AKJP-Heidelberg and/or held leadership positions there also benefited greatly from the complete lack of systematic organizational ethical discourse. The fact that in this way the harm of a large number of children, young adults and colleagues was accepted, could apparently be accepted with the help of the rationalization of the irrational.

As far as can be reconstructed, professional ethical issues have been recognizably represented at the Institute IPP-Heidelberg-Mannheim since at least the beginning of the 1990s. Seminars, lectures and conferences as well as corresponding initiatives of the umbrella organization DGPT contributed to the integration of professional ethical issues into the own organizational ethical context. With regard to AKJP-Heidelberg, the picture is somewhat different: After the partial exposure of the assaults of the institute director H. M. in 1993, the relationship to the umbrella association VAKJP was very strained. For many years, at least in parts of the AKJP-Heidelberg, there was a pronounced defensive attitude towards ethics-related impulses on the part of the VAKJP and the IPP-Heidelberg-Mannheim. Questions of professional and organizational ethics were contaminated for a long time by discrepant attitudes towards the "Causa H. M.". This was also related to the fact that persons were represented in leading committees of the AKJP-Heidelberg who had supported the organizational ethical failure of the AKJP-Heidelberg for many years and had also profited from it. When at the end of the 1990s the AKJP-Heidelberg called for the foundation of an ethics committee, this call was diverted – as far as this can be accurately reconstructed in retrospect – to the group "Past – Present – Future". It is interesting to note that the case of H. M. was discussed first and then the focus was on treatment-related issues and the Institute's public image. There is no sign here of any effort to establish an ethical position for the organization or to develop appropriate procedures and structures. Surprisingly, it was not until ten years later that two internal ethics officers were appointed. As far as can be seen, it was not until then that questions of professional ethics in particular were explicitly treated as such in the context of training. In addition, a systematic culture of reflection on organizational ethics seems to have developed since the events surrounding the court case against H. M. at the latest.

5.3 Abstinence

A specific variant of a professional ethical classification of the behaviour of the psychotherapist H. M. is opened up through references to psychoanalytical guiding concepts. Since the present study is concerned with the initiation of sexual relations in the psychotherapeutic setting, the following remarks focus on the concepts of "transference love" and "abstinence". With regard to the concept of abstinence, Kreische (1998) specifies that it is a technical principle "that demands the avoidance of transference gratifications, i.e. the refraining from fulfilling transference desires (…). Abstinence means abstinence. The abstinence principle demands abstinence from the analyst: He is to refrain from transference gratifications, even when the fulfillment of these wishes would please him himself" (p. 385). Based on these observations, it is important to differentiate the principle of abstinence from that of neutrality. According to Kreische (1998), abstinence is not to be understood as an aspect of neutrality, but the underlying dynamics of these two concepts are fundamentally different: "Neutrality in psychoanalytic treatment means that the analyst should keep his countertransference and his own transference to the patient under control, that he should avoid imposing his own values on the patient, and that he should use the patient's ability more than his own preferences as a guide to his actions" (p. 386). On the basis of these definitional foundations, the distinction could be made that the requirement of abstinence is aimed at more reactive processes, whereas neutrality addresses more the active motivations and intentions of the therapist. The starting point of the abstinence requirement is the therapist's countertransference feeling, which has its origin in the material that the patient presents in the context of psychotherapy. Neutrality, on the other hand, can much more easily be understood in terms of a principled "attitude" on the part of the therapist. Strictly speaking, the difference between these two concepts refers to assumptions about where the "actual" origin of sexual boundary violations lies in the psychotherapeutic setting. The abstinence requirement shifts this primarily to the patient, since in a narrower sense it is a "countertransference requirement". As a therapeutic attitude, the principle of neutrality, on the other hand, refers much more strongly to the possibility that a sexualization or eroticization of a therapeutic relationship could also be initiated "genuinely" on the part of the therapist. If one does not reduce the corresponding risks solely to the necessity of dealing responsibly with feelings of countertransference [as Freud, 1914 suggests], then the problem of sexual boundary violations in psychotherapy dealt with here would rather be subsumed under the term violation of neutrality. Accordingly, Kreische (1998) suspects a "defensive process" among psychoanalysts in the priority use of the term abstinence, "through which the perpetrator-victim relation is to be reversed or blurred" (p. 386).

In the present context, two case constellations are of particular interest, namely H. M.'s sexual relationships with young female patients and sexual relationships that he had with female students. By concentrating on those individual cases in which at least fragmentary information is available, it is not intended to re-stage that reductionism which obscured an accurate assessment of the events both in the phase of disclosure and for a long time afterwards. It should be noted, therefore, that a consideration of the context within which the sexual relationships with female patients and training candidates were initiated greatly simplifies the evaluation of those relationships. If we know that H. M. touched adolescent girls' breasts in the psychotherapeutic situation and invited them to further sexual acts, and if it is known that as the head of the institute he often maintained sexual relations with several training candidates at the same time, then this offers clear orientations regarding the genesis of that "love" which arose in the psychotherapies conducted by H. M.

In the psychoanalytic discourse on abstinence and transference love, one of the questions raised is how "strictly" the attitude of abstinence must be implemented in the psychotherapeutic setting, i.e. also how "neutrally" psychotherapists must behave towards the expressions, wishes and needs of their patients in order to achieve the therapeutic goals (e.g. Bauriedl, 1998; Pfannschmidt, 1998). Freud already pointed out in 1914 that the question of how to deal with "transference love" involves both ethical and treatment aspects (Freud, 1914). However, this is not so much a matter of making the doctor-patient* relationship compatible with bourgeois moral standards at all times, but rather the ethical obligation to abstinence stems from the fact that its non-consideration destroys the prospect of achieving therapeutic goals (Hirsch, 2012; Tschan, 2005). Long before psychoanalysis could evolve toward an "intersubjective turn," Freud located the emergence of feelings of love in psychotherapy solely in the optionally "sick," "neurotic," or "hysterical" patient. It is incumbent upon the physician to deal responsibly with the feelings of love brought into play by the patient. At this point it first becomes clear that this construction is only partially suitable for understanding what happened in H. M.'s psychotherapies. One might almost assume that Freud was unable to conceive of a "doctor" who actively and explicitly sexualized the psychotherapeutic situation from the very beginning. In any case, he started from different premises when he wrote that the doctor, to whom the patient's feelings of love refer, must realize "that the patient's falling in love is forced by the analytic situation and cannot be attributed, for instance, to the merits of his person, that he therefore has no reason at all to be proud of such a 'conquest' (…)" (Freud, 1914, p. 2). Here, the scene of therapeutically induced transference love is described, rather than the eroticization of the therapeutic relationship "forced" by the psychotherapist's offensive boundary violation. In fact, Freud's remarks are limited to such feelings of love that are brought into the therapeutic situation as a result of transference dynamics on the part of the patient. This corresponds to an understanding of "neutrality" from which the expression of biographically formed emotional impulses on the part of the psychotherapist is not envisaged. In fact, a fundamental paradigm shift in terms of an intersubjective understanding of the therapist-patient relationship was needed to allow for a systematic confrontation with the possibility that psychoanalytic therapies can also be contaminated by destructive desires and needs on the part of the therapist (Tibone & Schmieder-Dembek, 2015). Hirsch (2012) therefore comes to an assessment that diametrically contradicts that of Freud: "In the case of sexual boundary violation, it is usually not the patient at all, but the analyst or psychotherapist who sexualizes his own and at the same time also the patient's neediness and who introduces his gesture with sexuality (…)" (p. 55).

With regard to the case of H. M., much of what Freud writes in the remarks about "transference love" is nevertheless highly relevant, because it would have made possible a professional or professional-ethical evaluation of the facts that became known, even in ignorance of their origin. At this point, it should be recalled once again that in the course of the disclosures in 1992/1993, H. M. admitted that he had entered into sexual relations with two young female patients (namely, those who became pregnant by him) and three female teaching analysands allegedly *after the* completion of the therapies (or the "diagnostic conversations") and *after the* completion of the teaching analyses. Apart from the fact that these allegations are false, the question arises as to what Freud would have said about this "doctor." First of all, he would have started from the following outline of the problem: "If, then, the patient has fallen in love with the doctor, he will think, there can only be two outcomes, the rarer one that all circumstances permit the permanent legitimate union of the two, and the more frequent one that doctor and patient break up and abandon the work begun, which was to serve the production, as disturbed by an elementary event. Certainly a third outcome is also conceivable, which even seems to be compatible with the continuation of the cure, the establishment of illegitimate love relationships that are not destined for eternity; but this is probably made impossible by bourgeois morality as well as by medical dignity" (Freud, 1914, p. 2). As is well known, it became an identity-forming feature of psychoanalytic treatment that Freud described a fourth "exit" by declaring the feelings of infatuation to be an essential material of working through in the psychotherapeutic setting, with which special demands are made on the physician: "One is careful not to distract from the love transference, to scare it away, or to make the patient uncomfortable with it; one refrains just as steadfastly from any reciprocation of it" (ibid. p. 5). This is nothing other than the integration of transference love into a responsibly conducted therapeutic process, in the course of which the patient moves towards an increasingly free – i.e. freed from infantile fixations – disposal of her capacity for love, which she is not allowed to "spend in the cure" but which is to be "kept ready for real life" (ibid. p. 7). In order to achieve the therapeutic goals formulated here via the demanding path of working through erotic transference feelings, it is necessary to clearly define the role of the doctor: "The cure must be carried out in abstinence" (ibid. p. 5). And therefore "it is clear to him that he must derive no personal advantage from it [transference love, author's note]" (ibid. p. 7). Even if much of what Freud writes about the doctor-patient relationship seems anachronistic, he makes fundamental markings that are directly aimed at the ethical dimension of psychoanalytic action. The renunciation of reciprocating feelings of love in the context of psychoanalytic treatment does not follow the principles of a "bourgeois morality," but it provides a necessary framework for the fulfillment of the therapeutic mandate. The real love relationship and/or the real sexual act are therefore unethical not because they run counter to bourgeois moral concepts, but because the responsibility associated with any therapeutic treatment is thereby ignored on the part of the psychotherapist, thus accepting the continuation or exacerbation of damage to health (cf. Tschan, 2005). For "when the passions generated by the analytic process lead to aggressive-destructive or sexual acting out, when the framework is destroyed by action, psychoanalysis has a profoundly iatrogenic effect" (Krutzenbichler, 1998, p. 322). Therefore, "yielding remains out of the question for the analyst. As highly as he may value love, he must place the fact that he has the opportunity to lift his patient above a crucial stage in her life higher. She has to learn from him the overcoming of the pleasure principle, the renunciation of an obvious but socially unclassified satisfaction in favor of a more distant one, perhaps even uncertain, but psychologically as well as socially irreproachable" (Freud, 1914, p. 8).

Both the patients and the training analysands could have "learned" something from H. M. in this sense – and it should actually have been clear to everyone already at that time, when these relationships were eyed with more or less interest, that H. M. was depriving these women of those developmental potentials whose activation and expansion formed the original reason for their encounter. Pragmatically speaking, one can speak of "failed" psychotherapies and teaching analyses throughout. In order to better understand what happened, however, it makes sense to go beyond the basic orientation framework formulated by Freud and to consult contemporary discourses.

Since the 1980s at the latest, a large number of case reports and also empirical analyses have been published – especially in the US literature – dealing with the sexual exploitation of mostly female patients by mostly male psychotherapists (Celenza, 1991; Gabbard, 1994; Gartrell et al., 1987; Holroyd & Brodsky, 1977; Pope & Bouhoutsos, 1994; Rutter, 1990). This has led to a fundamental uncertainty among psychoanalysts about how to deal with erotic feelings and sexualized behaviour in the context of psychotherapy. The multitude of manifestations in this regard made differentiations necessary, especially since a comprehensive sensitization and scandalization with regard to sexual violence took place in many areas of society parallel to the psychoanalytic discourse (cf. Kavemann & Lohstöter, 1993). Hirsch (2012) refers to a variety of approaches to a terminological version of erotic or sexualized manifestations in the psychoanalytic setting and offers a distinction that seems to be profitable for our purposes: (1) *erotic-sexual* love (transference love), (2) erotized love, (3) (sadomasochistic-) perverted love.

In the sense of an improved understanding of the events surrounding H. M., we will navigate between the concepts proposed by Hirsch (2012), taking into account his "pattern of acts". This is done with the help of three concepts, to which a high explanatory value can be attributed for the classification of erotic-sexual manifestations in the psychotherapeutic setting: (1) Narcissistic love, (2) The boundary between fantasy and realization, (3) The ego boundaries of the patient.

5.3.1 Narcissistic Love

If we consider Freud's prohibition against deriving "personal advantage" from transference love, then in view of what we know about H. M.'s relationships with his patients and training analysands, it quickly becomes clear that transgressing this prohibition was a major motivation for the institute director's actions. In everything we learn about H. M. from his diaries and from conversations with people who knew him, an almost frightening degree of narcissistic neediness becomes apparent. It is readily demonstrable that he has been in an almost tragic, or at least compulsive, repetitive loop for decades, within which he uses the sexual exploitation of women for the temporary satisfaction of his narcissistic needs. In fact, the picture presented here is one of a repetition compulsion in the clinical sense. In the process, the psychotherapist is repeatedly euphorized by "actual" feelings of love, whereby what makes him happy here is not the relation with other people, but the at least temporarily abundant narcissistic gain. If one reads H. M.'s diaries, they provide a fairly accurate reflection of what Hirsch (2012) writes about the dynamics of narcissistic love: "The aging analyst hopes for the participation in his patient's youthfulness, or he sees qualities in her that he himself must miss and that he thinks he can add to his self through love and the union it brings. When two people in such narcissistic need meet, they each see what is lacking in the other and hope for self-supplementation, self-enhancement in a narcissistic collusion in the union of love" (p. 63). Very briefly, one could say that the narcissistic self-appreciation of female patients and teaching analysands consisted in being "chosen" by the respected doctor and institute director (which, for example, represents an unexpected psychological gain for a traumatized girl socialized in youth welfare).

For the aging psychotherapist, the profit of this narcissistic valorization consists in sexual self-assurance, which – according to the following remarks by Hirsch

(2012) – is equivalent to a self-assurance of the whole person: "The male body or, even more reduced, the male genitalia and its idolization ("admiration", acceptance) [are] supposed to compensate for a lack of self-esteem, a lack of a sense of identity (especially as a man). The analyst confuses his analytic competence, perhaps also (not necessarily!) his greater life experience with sexual potency, which has perhaps decreased in real terms over the years" (p. 91).

It is easily recognizable that H. M. entangles both his patients and his teaching analysands in a narcissistically motivated repetition compulsion, which is relatively uncomplicated to initiate: For both participants, the narcissistic gain from the sexualization of the relationship can be experienced quickly in each case. One can speak here of a regularly "induced love" that does not come close to having the character of a transference love, but functions as a potential concomitant of a narcissistically motivated sexualization of the therapeutic setting. Against this background, it really does not matter whether the sexual relationship began during or after the "official" termination of psychotherapy or teaching analysis, because one will be able to claim with some justification that – in the sense of psychoanalytic treatment guidelines – there was no therapy and no teaching analysis at all.

5.3.2 The Line Between Fantasy and Realization

The psychoanalytical discussion on the question whether erotic feelings on the part of the psychotherapist towards his/her patient are "allowed" can basically be declared obsolete with regard to the "Causa H. M.". In this discussion, confusion is sometimes created with the argument that the psychoanalytic treatment technique is robbed of its substance if the emergence of such feelings is frowned upon from the outset or at least regarded as suspect (cf. Bittner, 1998). Such arguments can be refuted relatively easily with reference to Freud, since transference love and corresponding countertransference feelings are part of the usual repertoire of psychoanalytic treatment. This means that the fact that psychotherapists feel feelings of love towards their patients is neither ethically reprehensible nor an indication of a treatment error. The crucial question is rather how such feelings are "worked with" (Hirsch, 2012; Pfannschmidt, 1998). Whereas Freud held that transference and countertransference love are not "real" love feelings because they stem from past conflict-free love relationships, Hirsch (2012), citing Krutzenbichler and Essers (1991), argues that love feelings that emerge in the psychotherapeutic situation are "real" in character. At this point, the criterion of the "legitimacy" of such feelings manifests itself in the distinction between fantasy/desire on the one hand and "the acting out of such desires into reality" (Hirsch, 2012, p. 65) on the other. Here it is worth recalling all that Freud said in the "Remarks on Transference Love" about the psychoanalytic treatment technique and the mechanisms underlying its effectiveness (Freud, 1914). The emotional reality of the feeling of love constitutes the "material" for therapeutic treatment, which is nullified the moment the urge for real (sexual) consummation of this feeling is yielded to. Hirsch (2012) therefore stresses the importance of "restrictive barriers" that must be maintained "between thinking, speaking, fantasizing on the one hand and doing, acting, and acting on on the other hand" (ibid. p. 68).[5] Fundamental, therefore, is the analyst's ability "to fantasize, to play through wishes and impulses mentally first and not to have to put them into action right away" (ibid. p. 68).

The only thing that can be credited to H. M. in this context is the fact that he did not always have to put his narcissistically motivated sexual desire into action "immediately". It must be noted, however, that the ability to draw a clear line between symbolizing and acting, which is crucial for the success of the psychoanalytic treatment, was obviously underdeveloped. The extent to which he deliberately created the impression of having been "seduced" by the patients and teaching analysands is irrelevant, since it was his responsibility to ensure that the boundary between desire and action was not crossed under any circumstances.

5.3.3 The Ego Limits of Female Patients

Hirsch (2012) explicitly emphasizes this latter aspect of the assignment of responsibility: "Even if the complementarity and collusion between the analyst's narcissistic needs of exploitation and the patient's illusionary longing for a father, who both hope to heal the narcissistic wound through sexuality, must be acknowledged, the responsibility to prevent the acting out of the desires always lies with the therapist" (p. 130). To make clear the destructive character of an acted sexualization in the psychotherapeutic setting, Hirsch (2012) argues by means of the identity theory: the patient comes to psychotherapy seeking for help or, in transference, as a child in need of protection and care. In doing so, she exposes herself to dependency vis à vis the psychotherapist, "for the arrangement of psychoanalytic therapy (…), in which the patient is supposed to reveal himself entirely, to open up, while the analyst communicates nothing about himself, creates an asymmetry: the analyst keeps out his own emotional areas, reacting instead with the help of the so-called

[5] Körner (1998b) derives precisely from this the special responsibility of psychotherapists with regard to the level of action: "Because we are allowed to fantasize everything, we must be all the more certain about the limits of our action" (p. 299).

countertransference in a professionally controlled and reflected way to the emotions of the patient, who is now supposed to open up entirely" (p. 163). It is immediately evident that through the regression-promoting setting described here, an increased vulnerability with regard to the patient's ego limits is "structurally inherent"[6] (cf. Bauriedl, 1998). In order for the patient to maintain her "identity as a patient," it is of substantial importance that her ego boundaries be maintained. The moment the analyst sexualizes the therapeutic relationship and releases the feelings of love from the symbolic level of desire into the real (sexual) consummation, the patient loses her identity as a patient. She is, so to speak, deprived of her right to be a patient and to seek help. Or to put it another way: The patient's ego boundaries are violated to such an extent that she ceases to exist as a patient (just as the student can no longer exist as a student when her teacher sexualizes the relationship; just as the daughter can no longer exist as a daughter when her father sexualizes the relationship).

In the case of H. M. it can be clearly stated that both patients and teaching analysands were robbed of their identity with which they came into contact with H. M. This means that the moment the relationship became sexual, the patients no longer received any help and the teaching analysands no longer received any teaching analysis. This means that the moment the relationship became sexual, the patients no longer received any help and the teaching analysands no longer received any teaching analysis. The consequences for the women exploited in this way were correspondingly severe (see Becker-Fischer & Fischer, 1996; Burka, 2008; Wallace, 2007). Female patients and teaching analysands became mistresses of the doctor and institute director. The narcissistic gain associated with this very soon left behind an emptiness that was difficult to bear – and the regular realization that,

[6] "In psychotherapeutic treatment, certain functions of a patient which, from a developmental-psychological point of view, are restricted, handicapped or missing, are promoted so that they can mature. In order to be able to achieve such a psychological change, a loosening of the psychological structures and thus an at least partial regression are necessary, which are accompanied by a partial loss of autonomy. These changes are promoted and made possible with the pressure of suffering on the part of the patient. On the other hand, the aforementioned restricted functions as well as the regressive processes with loosening of intrapsychic structures also make a mentally ill patient particularly vulnerable and susceptible (…)" Schleu et al. (2018, p. 14).

at some point, she was neither a patient/teaching analysand nor H. M.'s lover made the pain of the deeply violated boundaries of the ego palpable in its full extent.[7]

The considerations made here point to the importance of fundamental psychoanalytic concepts in relation to the design of psychotherapeutic settings in general. Without being able to even approximately depict the discourse in this regard at this point, it is nevertheless recognizable that attention to transference-countertransference dynamics and ongoing reflexive self-assurance are elementary with regard to psychotherapeutic attitudes and psychotherapeutic action. A consideration of the "Causa H. M." in the mirror of psychoanalytically founded concepts leads to the insight that this is an extreme case. The attempt made everywhere to conceptualize his offenses as "abstinence violations" seems euphemistic at first. However, this labelling enables an appropriate professional ethical orientation, which can function as a basis for consequences in the sense of at least professionally justifiable sanctions (Tibone & Schmieder-Dembek, 2015). In retrospect, it can be stated that for a long time everything that could be effectively argued against H. M. was argued with recourse to the concept of abstinence violation. This insight is important because neither criminal law nor moral outrage allowed for comparatively sustained interventions (Molitor, 1998). Not everything had to be known in order to nevertheless be able to prove the abstinence violations to an extent that led to his resignation as head of the institute, his withdrawal from the psychoanalytic umbrella organizations, and at least a local restriction of his work as an expert witness.

In the overall view, however, it becomes clear that H. M. was by no means moving in a "borderline area" of abstinence violation. This borderline area is the one around which diverse discussions are grouped within the psychoanalytic scene (Bittner, 1998; Hirsch, 2012). This is where, for example, the question of how long the "latency period" after a completed psychotherapy must last in order to be able to enter into a "legitimate" love relationship between psychotherapist and patient can be located (Schleu et al., 2018). There are different positions on this in the

[7] This is reminiscent of a case described by Schleu et al. (2018): "Initially, the patient's longing is ignited by the psychotherapist, she is "fed" recognition (…) and seduced into secret closeness and intimacy. In the further course, however, the abusive relationship is abruptly terminated because the concealment is no longer successful. The psychotherapist accepts the loss of the supposed love without suffering himself, but for the patient an illusory world collapses with the corresponding damaging consequences: psychological breakdown with confusion and inability to act, loss of personal relationships, social isolation, inability to work, severe depressive disorders requiring treatment, up to suicidal tendencies" (p. 18).

various psychoanalytic associations.[8] The attempt to reduce the "Causa H. M." to such questions amounts to a deliberate argumentative confusion, which was actively pursued by himself and his allies. Even though diagnostic statements are not part of the investigation at hand here, all available information suggests that H. M. is a "repeat offender of the sexually perverted type" (Hirsch, 2012). This attribution imposes itself when we consider the following outline of the motivations underlying sexual boundary violations (Wirtz 1989; cited in Hirsch, 2012, p. 91): "After all, sexual assaults in therapy are often not primarily about sexuality, and even less about love and therapy, but about the addictive search for validation, the lack of an internalized sense of being accepted, or the savoring of power in a dependent relationship." When dealing with such offenders, the question naturally no longer arises as to whether the sexual relationship began during or after therapy. Nor does the question arise as to whether there was therapy or only diagnostic discussions, or during what period of time after the completion of therapy the sexual relationship was initiated. And the assumption that marriage legitimizes a relationship thus formed can presumably only be voiced by those who rely on improvised self-soothing in the face of their failures and misperceptions.

The following remarks from H. M.'s diary substantiate the classification made here. They provide clues to his social neediness as well as to the fact that he apparently did not even spare himself with the manipulative legitimation of his sexual boundary violations:

"When a woman as a patient sits in front of me or lies on the couch for years, telling me her worries, her disappointments, her longings, her entire life fate, then an extremely intimate, personal relationship develops, which as a rule is more

---

[8] See, for example, the sample professional code of conduct of the Federal Chamber of Psychotherapists of 10.11.2007, §6 (7): "The abstinence requirement also applies to the period after the end of psychotherapy, as long as there is still a need for treatment or a relationship of dependence between the patient and the psychotherapist. The responsibility for a professionally ethical procedure lies solely with the treating psychotherapist. Before private contacts are initiated, a time interval of at least 1 year must be observed."

The ethical guidelines of the DGPT (version of 23.09.2011) state: "In particular, he [the psychotherapist, author's note] does not enter into sexual relationships with patients/analysts. He respects the abstinence requirement even beyond the termination of the analytic working relationship."

In the "Ethical Principles of Psychologists and Code of Conduct" of the American Psychological Association (APA) of 1.1.2017 the following strict regulation is set: "Psychologists do not engage in sexual intimacies with former clients/patients for at least 2 years after cessation or termination of therapy". Even after 2 years of "latency period", the establishment of a sexual relationship between psychotherapist and former patient is only possible under very specific conditions.

intense than relationships as they develop in ordinary life. The so-called transference love from the patient to the therapist, described by Freud, frequently arises, much as it does in ordinary life. Very often women marry men who resemble their fathers or brothers, men look for mothers or sisters in their wives. The countertransference love from the therapist to the patient during an analysis develops equally intensely toward such people as those that one might fall in love with in ordinary life. That I was particularly susceptible was not least due to the fact that after moving to Heidelberg, in 1975, I no longer had a steady partner and had always avoided social events where I could have met women. My co-workers, my patients and female patients were my social connections! This became my downfall. It's easy to get morally indignant about this weakness, but this specific situation of a long-term analysis, which only succeeds when an intense familiarity has developed, can really only be judged by someone who has experienced it himself."

5.4 Sexual Violence

As we have seen, a conceptual location of H. M.'s sexual boundary violations in a professional-ethical context is meaningful and necessary, but cannot remain there. In view of the multitude of sexual boundary violations and the – as far as is known – serious consequences for the victims, the labeling as "abstinence violation" tends to seem trivializing. It is therefore important, in the sense of a precise conceptual definition of the phenomena examined here, to approach them from a field of discourse that is not genuinely psychotherapeutic but has its origins in a sociopolitically motivated scandalization of the sexual exploitation of girls and women in the 1970s/1980s. The discourse, which was originally primarily based on feminism, has since undergone various differentiations, but is ultimately still traceable to those essential basic concepts through which the topic of "sexual exploitation" experienced a linguistic representation (Maurer, 2018).

In the context of H. M., a conceptualization related to these discourses is not easy, since we are dealing with very heterogeneous constellations of acts and actions. This becomes immediately evident when we contrast the request to a 6-year-old to undress in the examination room with a sexual relationship with a teaching analysand that lasted for years. What are we dealing with here? In the following, we will make a few determinations of where we stand, which are of an orientational character and should contribute to a terminological classification of what is happening.

If we first look at the sexual boundary violations committed by H. M. towards boys and girls in the examinations, then a reference to a well-known definition by

Bange and Deegener (1996) suggests itself: "Sexual abuse of children is any sexual act that is performed on or in front of a child either against the child's will or to which the child cannot knowingly consent due to physical, psychological, cognitive or linguistic inferiority. The perpetrator uses his position of power and authority to satisfy his own needs at the expense of the child" (p. 96). Taking into account the stipulation formulated here, it seems legitimate and accurate to describe all of H. M.'s sexual acts towards boys and girls in the context of psychotherapies and second sights as sexual abuse. What he was only proven to have done "ex officio" in 2017 in connection with his granddaughter, he had previously practiced for decades with an unknown number of children. From a criminal law perspective, such acts are covered by sections 176[9] and 176a of the Criminal Code. In this context, it must be taken into account that, due to the developmental psychological aspects described above, there can be no consensual sexual acts between children and adults. This means that even a superficial "cooperation" of boys and girls during the examination does not change the fact that the offence of sexual abuse is fulfilled. Ignorant of the legal argumentations that led to the respective discontinuation of the two criminal proceedings against H. M. (1995 and 2013) for sexual abuse of children known to us, it can be assumed that in the second case (2013) the statute of limitations had expired, while in the first case presumably those legitimation strategies were applied that were available to H. M. for all such cases: Insignificance of the crime, medically justified necessity of the examination practices. It can also be assumed that no defined code was available to the investigating authorities as to what a delegation doctor may and may not do in the context of the psychoanalytically based second sight The doctor should not have found it difficult to make a plausible association of the sexual with the psychoanalytic. The definition by Bange and Deegener (1996), published only a year later, could have provided valuable insights in this regard: "The perpetrator exploits his position of power and authority to satisfy his own needs at the expense of the child".

In contrast to sexual acts between adults and children (under 14 years of age), sexual acts between adults and adolescents are only punishable under certain conditions, which primarily relate to the demonstrable exploitation of the lack of capacity for sexual self-determination on the part of the adolescent (Section 182 of the Criminal Code). A criminal sanctionability of the sexual assaults demonstrably committed by H. M. against – primarily female – juvenile patients can be assumed as a rule, however, from today's perspective, no assessments can be made about the

[9] § Section 176 of the Criminal Code, subsection (1): "Whoever performs sexual acts on a person under fourteen years of age (child) or has such acts performed on him by the child shall be punished by imprisonment for a term of 6 months to 10 years."

legal practice at that time in such cases. In any case, §174c would apply here, which refers to sexual abuse in the context of psychotherapy. In the specific case, this would affect all those offences committed from 1998 onwards. But even before 1998, criminal sanctioning would have been possible via the offence of sexual coercion.

Sections 174a, b and c StGB refer to the fact that the term sexual abuse does not only refer to sexual acts towards minors. These laws regulate sexual abuse of adults in different dependency relationships (e.g. in prisons, care relationships,…). Since it is of central importance for the context examined here, §174c, para. 2 is reproduced in its wording:

> §174c Sexual abuse taking advantage of a counseling, treatment, or supervisory relationship:
>
> (2) A person who performs sexual acts on a person entrusted to him for psychotherapeutic treatment, or causes them to be performed on him, in abuse of the treatment relationship, shall also be punished.

Since this legal provision was only introduced in 1998, it could not apply to the cases of sexual relations with adult female patients and teaching analysts that have come to our attention in more detail. The requirement of "abuse of the treatment relationship" would also have raised the threshold of argumentation for any plaintiffs. It should be noted, however, that possible starting points for criminal sanctions were available through the criminal offences of rape or sexual assault (which are associated with threats, the use of force or the exploitation of a coercive situation).

It becomes clear that although the criminal law offers important conceptual orientations and also options for action, it is, on the other hand, only insufficiently suitable for recording the different forms of sexual exploitation and, above all, also for providing reliable sanctions[10] (Schleu et al., 2018).

[10] The question of the criminal sanctioning of sexual transgressions within the framework of psychoanalysis was the subject of controversial discussions at a conference of the DGPT in 1997. One line of argumentation consisted – formulated in a simplified way – in the fact that it is problematic if the solution of conflicts and dynamics arising in the course of the psychoanalytic process is delegated to the outside, i.e. to state authorities. Pfannschmidt (1998) formulates a very pointed metaphor for this problem: "Anyone who allows a fire to occur in his house, which he cannot control himself, must tolerate and also be satisfied with the fire brigade kicking in the doors so that they can extinguish it. The fact that the damage caused by extinguishing is often quite considerable has never been an argument for not extinguishing" (p. 371).

Around the turn of the millennium, the term "sexual violence" began to establish itself in the professional discussion, which relates the event in question more strongly to the feelings of the victim and relates the dynamics of the event in question primarily to a sexualization of power relations.[11] Retkowski et al. (2018) locate this conceptualization as the result of a longer history of discourse. In their view, the term "sexual violence" addresses the "structural, discursive, symbolic aspect of violence as well as institutional and organizational relations of violence" (p. 23). With the help of this term, the perspective on „structural and institutionalized relations of inequality as enabling conditions for sexual violence" (ibid. p. 23) is reinforced. In this way, the conceptual horizon is broadened, which clearly points beyond the criminal act of "sexual abuse". Nevertheless, there is something ambivalent about the term "sexual violence": On the one hand, it expresses the destructive character of every sexual boundary violation, while at the same time it obscures the view of everything that is perceived as "non-violent" by the victims or other persons who have knowledge of such cases. What is at stake here is the problem of different subjective representations of the concept of violence, which comes to the fore in connection with "love relationships" between the director of the institute and female students of teaching analysis that have lasted for years, just as it does in the case of the request to the child presented for second sight to undress. In any case, there is room for interpretation here that cannot be resolved simply by declaring certain actions on the part of "authorized" parties to be violence.

Enders et al. (2010) offer a differentiation that is particularly important for pedagogical practice with the help of the terms "assaults" and "boundary violations that are committed unintentionally". Criteria for the classification of corresponding acts are above all the frequency of occurrence as well as the responsiveness or reflectiveness with regard to one's own behaviour on the part of the person who initiated the acts. This opens up useful starting points for psychotherapy, as "unintentional boundary violations" can also occur in the psychotherapeutic setting, which cannot be categorized as sexual assault or sexual abuse. Such boundary violations are possibly to be placed in the conceptual vicinity of abstinence violations, which can manifest themselves in non-sexual physical touching or questions perceived as unpleasant (in the sense of "transgressing"). In distinction to this, sexual assault is an intentional offence, which, however, is still below the threshold of criminal sanctionability. The shameful conversations and questioning that H. M. conducted with his patients can be cited here as an example.

---

[11] The term "sexual violence" is currently finding its way into the legal discourse for the first time in connection with the "Draft Law to Combat Sexual Violence against Children" (see https://www.bundestag.de/presse/pressemitteilungen/pm-201202-recht-gewalt-kinder-811100)

It becomes clear that well-founded differentiations provide an important basis for adequate professional reactions to "conspicuous behaviour", since not every boundary violation can be qualified as "abuse" or "sexual violence" and corresponding misjudgements can lead to overreactions on the one hand or failures on the other. Furthermore, it is important to note that affected persons often only „get an idea "of what was inflicted on them in an earlier phase of their lives in the course of their biography (Draucker & Martsolf, 2008; Kavemann et al. 2015a; Keupp et al., 2019; Rieske et al., 2018). The love affair with the head of the institute or the psychotherapist or the strange experience at the pediatrician's office can often only be fitted years later into a conceptual structure that corresponds much more closely to one's own emotional feelings than the powerful manipulative narrative of the perpetrator (who was not recognizable as such at the time) (Unabhängige Aufarbeitungskommission, 2017). The linguistic marking of events that often took place in secret and were subject to the interpretive power of a single person is therefore of particular importance (Draucker & Martsolf, 2008).

The analysis of the "Causa H. M." makes it possible, at least retrospectively, to determine the corresponding position, whereby the terminology used is partially oriented towards criminal law, but naturally does not involve a judicially secured determination:

The sexual acts towards children (under 14 years of age) in second sights and psychotherapies that have become known to us allow a classification as sexual abuse of children.

Assaults against adolescents in the context of second sights and psychotherapies qualify as sexual abuse of adolescents, sexual assault or sexual coercion.

All sexual acts that involved adult female patients and teaching analysts would now be sanctioned as sexual abuse taking advantage of a treatment relationship.

H. M. acted intentionally, taking into account the embarrassment and/or the violation of the physical and psychological integrity of the minors and adults to whom the sexualizations initiated by him referred. A final consideration of the individual constellations of offences justifies the application of the term "sexual violence" to all cases that have come to our attention, since H. M. at all times made use of the structural and institutional inequalities that he helped to create (Retkowski et al., 2018) in order to help his personal needs to prevail. As institute director, physician, psychotherapist, teaching analyst, and supervisor, he always initiated the sexualization of interactions and relationships from the position of the powerful. It could be objected that the application of the term "sexual violence" to all sexual acts of persons between whom there is an imbalance of power is excessive. In the case of H. M., however, this objection cannot be asserted, since he fundamentally and in constant repetition made use of his position of power in order to obtain sexual arousal towards children, adolescents and young women.

(Sexual) Boundary Violations in Psychotherapeutic Relationships: An Inventory

6

> *The cure must be carried out in abstinence; I do not mean by this the physical deprivation alone, nor the deprivation of all that one desires, for perhaps no sick person would tolerate this. But I want to establish the principle that need and longing must be allowed to exist in the sick as forces driving them to work and change, and that one must be careful not to appease them by surrogates. One could not offer anything other than surrogates, since the sick person, as a result of her condition, is incapable of real satisfaction as long as her repressions have not been remedied.* (Freud, 1949 [1914], p. 313)

H. M. was and is not an isolated case. As a cursory glance at the relevant literature shows, the topic of boundary violations was discussed early on in the psychoanalytic community, as the example of the relationship between Sabina Spielrein and C. G. Jung at the beginning of the twentieth century shows. A more intensive debate emerged in the 1990s, also in connection with women's political discussions about (male) violence and power, which found its echo in the psychotherapeutic professional public and in the media public and finally resulted in a reform of criminal law. In 1998, §174 c, Para. 2 StGB (the German Penal Code) was introduced, which made it possible to legally sanction sexual acts in psychotherapeutic

P. Caspari et al., *At some point there has to be peace and quiet!*,
https://doi.org/10.1007/978-3-658-39785-2_6

relationships and counselling.[1] After the punishability of sexual acts was enshrined in the code, the public discussion initially died down again.

Already in Freud's time, boundary violations in psychotherapeutic situations were discussed. The so-called abstinence rule has undergone changes over the years, and has been interpreted and discussed differently in the various directions of the differentiating psychoanalysis. The core of the abstinence rule is undisputed: sexual relations between therapists and patients during therapy are taboo. Erotic activity in the Freudian sense leads to a dissolution of the therapeutic relationship and transforms it into an everyday relationship (cf. Bossi, 1994, p. 45).

Nevertheless, boundary violations in psychotherapeutic relationships have occurred and continue to occur. For a long time, however, this was not a topic outside a limited professional public. Bossi (1994, p. 47) suspects that this is due to a special collective repression of sexual contacts with dependants, which could also apply to other dependency relationships. This collective repression can in any case be confirmed with regard to former children in institutions, boarding school children and/or children and adolescents in church contexts.[2] Here, public disclosure or inquiryonly began around 2010 and only through pressure from victims.

With regard to boundary violations in psychotherapeutic relationships, an initial discussion began in the 1980s in the USA. The first empirical data provided an inkling of the extent. Various regional and national studies conducted in the USA between 1968 and 1990 showed that between 4.8% and 17% of male therapists had sexual contact with patients. Female therapists were included in only two studies. Here, between 0.6 and 3.5% of the respondents reported sexual contact with patients (Bossi, 1994, p. 49f.).

---

[1] §174c as amended 11.4.2004 Sexual abuse taking advantage of a counselling, treatment or care relationship.

1. Any person who performs sexual acts on a person entrusted to him or her for counselling, treatment or care on account of a mental or psychological illness or disability, including an addictive disease, or on account of a physical illness or disability, or who has such acts performed on him or her, abusing the counselling, treatment or care relationship, shall be liable to a custodial sentence of 3 months to 5 years.

2. Any person who performs sexual acts on a person entrusted to him or her for psychotherapeutic treatment, or has such acts performed on him or her, in abuse of the treatment relationship, shall also be punished.

3. The attempt is punishable.

In the version of 1.4.1998, the phrase "or because of a physical illness or disability" was still missing. In addition, a fine was still possible in this first version. This was deleted in 2004.

[2] Cf. the working through the past studies of the IPP Munich: Keupp et al. (2017a, b, 2019), Caspari et al. (2021).

In the German-speaking psychotherapy scene, these results led to an intensive discourse that lasted until the end of the 1990s. Here, a circle of female therapists from the German Society for Behaviour Therapy (DGVT) was particularly active, the working group "Women in Psychotherapeutic Care". In 1991, a public hearing was held in Bonn with the title "Sexual Assault in Therapy. Malpractice or trivial offence?", which initiated a broader discussion of the topic. Empirical research on this field also began in Germany in the 1990s. Here, the work of Monika Becker-Fischer and Gottfried Fischer should be mentioned above all, who in 1993 began to investigate epidemiological and forensic psychological aspects of sexual assault in psychotherapy and psychiatry on behalf of the Federal Ministry for Family Affairs, Senior Citizens, Women and Youth. In 1996 the volume "Sexual abuse in psychotherapy – what to do? Orientation aids for therapists and interested patients" (Becker-Fischer & Fischer, 1996), which contained both an overview of the state of art and the data as well as information on possibilities for help for victims. The publication was based on a study for the Federal Ministry for Family Affairs, Senior Citizens, Women and Youth (Becker-Fischer & Fischer, 1995) and provided a data basis for Germany for the first time.

The IPP-Heidelberg-Mannheim also participated in the discourse. Around 1995 a panel took place, whose contributions appeared in issue 12/1995 of the institute's journal "Psychoanalysis in Contradiction". In the preface the then director of the institute wrote: "The fashionable topic of sexual abuse has also reached in the form of serious abstinence violations our institute. (…) The events have shown us that a psychoanalytic institution in its reactions or conscious and unconscious defence mechanisms is in no way different from usual family and accompanying social structures. Consciously not wanting to perceive, fear of shame, denial, defamation, pressure on the victims, formal legal threats, and above all the attempt to make the victims and those who name the abuse the actual perpetrators have become experiences of our institute" (Psychoanalyse im Widerspruch, 13/95). In these brief sentences, triggered by the dynamics in the IPP-Heidelberg-Mannheim, the defense mechanisms of the guild are clearly named.

In the early days of the discussion, the focus was rather less on the victims or the health consequences for them. Freud already suggests that it is a certain clinical picture that favours the love of the (female) patient for the (male) therapist: hysteria. For Freud, transference love seemingly takes place only in the heterosexual space and is directed from the patient to the therapist. The concept of countertransference was elaborated by Freud somewhat later.

In the case of transference love, the doctor must react professionally, must reflect and must not succumb to love if he does not want to endanger the "cure".

> *The analytic psychotherapist has thus to wage a threefold struggle, within himself against the powers which would like to drag him down from the analytic level, outside the analysis against the opponents who deny him the importance of the sexual instinctive forces and refuse to allow him to make use of them in his scientific technique, and in the analysis against his patients, who at first behave like the opponents, but then make known the overestimation of sexual life which dominates them and want to imprison the doctor with their socially unbridled passion.* (Freud, 1949 [1914], p. 320)

The renewed debate in the USA and later in Germany also initially focused on patient participation.

> *A particular danger to the analyst's abstinence attitude arises when working with patients in whom there is a structural ego disturbance, a pregenital disturbance, a structure that necessitates variations in technique.* (Cremerius, 1988; quoted in Heyne, 1991)

From various studies and surveys, a kind of psychopathology of the patients was developed. According to this, especially borderline patients were at risk. Also victims of sexual abuse within the family, for whom four factors were identified that predispose them to a repetition of the abuse experience:

> serious psychopathological disorders (…), idiosyncratic dynamics, atypical socialization or neglect, below-average cognitive problem-solving level, especially as a result of emotional neglect (Bossi, 1994, p. 60).

In this context, Bossi points out that such data are often misinterpreted – both in the psychotherapeutic community and in jurisprudence – by assigning patients a share of the blame. Or, in other words, the responsibility of the therapist is diminished.

Ursula Wirtz argued similarly. "The inability to draw a clear line to the idealized therapist, the inability to say 'no' is then falsely interpreted as an adult 'yes', as a voluntary consent to sexual contact. The apparent voluntariness virtually characterizes the typical scenario of an abuse of dependence and trust" (Wirtz, 1994, p. 40).

In contrast, Becker-Fischer and Fischer were able to show in their studies that in 78% of cases the initiative for sexual contact came from the therapist (Becker-Fischer & Fischer, 1995, p. 43). In the 2006 follow-up study, the figure was 80%. "This was usually not a sudden, unmediated assault, but the sexual contact was prepared by subtle means" (Becker-Fischer & Fischer, 2018, p. 61). According to the authors, this included small boundary violations, favours, private meetings such as visits to restaurants, the disclosure of his personal difficulties on the part of the therapist or sensitivities.

The Role of the Women's Movement

Especially women who were active in the women's movement and in psychotherapeutic professional associations made abuse in psychotherapy a topic in the 1990s and transferred it into a (professional) political discourse about power and dependencies. This brought the debate to focus in the public perception of sexual boundary violations, on abstinence violations between male therapists and adult female patients. Male victims barely featured in the literature. Female perpetrators on the margins. The focus of interest was on heterosexual relationships and orientations, both on the side of the therapists and on the side of the female patients. Underage female patients were not the subject of scientific or professional interest. Bossi only cites one study in which surprising data on the age and gender of the patients can be found:

> *Bajit (1989) found that a majority of the patients with whom therapists engaged in sexual contact were minors. Slightly more than half of these were female. Ages varied from 3 to 17 years for girls and from 7 to 16 years for boys. The average age was 13 for girls and 12 for boys. Furthermore, we do not have any studies that can provide detailed information about the age of patients with sexual experiences in the context of therapeutic relationships.* (Bossi, 1994, p. 53)[3]

This exception does not change the fact that the discussion of sexual boundary violations in psychotherapeutic relationships in the 1990s is embedded in the women's political discourse of the time about (male) power and the resulting (female) dependencies. In this respect, the debate of the 1990s reproduces the narrowing to heterosexual relationships among adults that was already evident in Freud.

> *We will be fundamentally at risk of becoming victims of sexual violence – quite regardless of our particular history – as long as men persist in asserting their claims to power over us women by using sexuality as a means of destruction.* (Heyne, 1991, p. 150)

This line of argumentation is well documented in the public hearing "Sexual Assault in Therapy. Malpractice or trivial offence?", which was organized in 1991 by the DGVT together with the Paritätischer Wohlfahrtsverband (Vogt, 1991).

[3] This "abstinence" of research towards the question of boundary violations against children and adolescents in therapeutic settings continues up to the present day. There are hardly any studies on this topic. In 2006 Fegert deals with sexual abuse by professionals in institutions (not in outpatient therapy situations) and sees a structural problem in the fact that the closeness in care relationships carries the risk of exploitation through an asymmetrical power relationship (Fegert, 2006).

This set the public debate in motion, albeit initially in a politically legitimate narrowing to adult women as victims. The attempts at uncovering in connection with the AKJP-Heidelberg and H. M. as perpetrator documented above are embedded in this discourse.

However, little attention has been paid to the involvement of training candidates and/or teaching analysts, even though they are in a special relationship of dependency. Bossi makes some references to studies from the USA in the 1980s. According to these, between 1.6% and 23% of students/trainees had sexual contact with their teachers or therapists or analysts. The majority of these relationships began early in training, and some led to later marriages. The question posed by the researchers at the time as to whether therapists who had sexual contact with their instructors during their training were more likely to engage in boundary violations with their own patients later on could not be answered satisfactorily. Further consequences for the candidates were not discussed (Bossi, 1994, p. 60f.).

In the panel of the IPP-Heidelberg-Mannheim, too, there are no contributions on this particular dependency, but there is one remark. In her contribution, Maier-Kirstätter asks about the "gap" that also remained in the IPP-Heidelberg-Mannheim when it was revealed: "What had actually happened? (…) This question could not be answered considering the best interest of the women victims. There remained a gap (…) and I encountered in myself (…) an inability, which at first seemed strange to me, to develop fantasies about this question, what really happened. (…) In retrospect I think this inability did not overcome me so much as a therapist, nor as a woman, but as an analysand with a teaching analyst and as a candidate for training" (Maier-Kirstätter, 1995, p. 7).

The broader questions that arose from this remained (and remain) unanswered. Is it a different form of concern when a sexual/intimate relationship develops between an almost-ready colleague and a teaching analyst? Can this be undone by marriage after training? What additional relationships of power and dependency are victims under? And how have they been prepared for their work as a psychotherapist?

Offender Profiles

There are various qualitative and quantitative studies on perpetrator profiles from the USA and also from German-speaking countries in the 1990s. Becker-Fischer and Fischer report on a perpetrator typology that was obtained based on many years of experience in the treatment of "affected female patients and transgressive therapists" (Becker-Fischer & Fischer, 2018). The American clinicians Schoener, Milgrom and Luepker identified six offender types:

1. Uninformed Naive. This includes mainly semi-professional therapists with little training and little personal maturity.
2. Healthy or average neurotic. This group includes one-time offenders who recognize their responsibility and want to work through the "case".
3. Severely neurotic and/or socially isolated. This group of therapists has clear emotional problems themselves, which they want to compensate for through therapeutic work.
4. Impulsive character disorders. This type includes therapists with difficulties in drive control. They have usually committed boundary violations prior to their therapeutic work. These therapists usually have sexual contacts with many female patients, simultaneously or consecutively. They only show guilt when they are threatened with consequences.
5. Sociopathic or narcissistic character disorders. Therapists from this group are experts in seducing patients and covering up these acts to colleagues.
6. Psychotic or borderline personalities. This group has only weak social judgment. Their sense of reality is disturbed.

According to Schoener et.al., the prognosis for successful rehabilitation is only given in group 2 (cited in Becker-Fischer & Fischer, 2018, p. 45ff)

Bossi, citing Twemlow and Gabbard (1989), reports three types of offenders: the psychopaths, the psychotics and the lovesick (Bossi, 1994, p. 55). Again, only the last type has a positive prognosis.

Hirsch sees a danger especially in the repeat offenders: "…repeat offenders who, due to their perverse personality and in an addictive manner, repeatedly seduce patients. Usual laws and guidelines for dealing with attraction do not concern them anyway because of general rule breaking" (Hirsch, 2018, p. 87).

These findings initially led to demands for improved training.

Professional Policy Considerations

In the development of the psychotherapeutic profession, elements can be found that are based on the historically developed professions. In sociology, the term profession is understood to mean a specific type of professionalism that requires an academic education and is associated with various privileges. Classical professions were medicine, theology, jurisprudence (cf. Stichweh, 2005; Pfadenhauer & Sander, 2010), which in the European tradition go back to the society of estates.

> *Historically, the concept of profession means a particular form of professionalism that has come to modern society from the class-corporate world of ancient Europe. Examples were first the academic professions of theologian, lawyer and physician,*

which found their place of training in the faculties of the medieval and early modern university. (...) The social status of the professions was extraordinarily high. They embodied the form in which, through professionalism, one could attain a social rank that was otherwise only accessible by birth through nobility. (...) Institutionally, the professions were organized corporately. They thus embodied the form of structural formation that had been taking its place alongside the status since the late Middle Ages. Corporations were permitted and privileged by ecclesiastical and secular powers. (Stichweh, 2005, p. 1f)

For psychotherapy, the alignment with medicine as a leading profession was advantageous, as it led to psychoanalytic treatment being billable as a health insurance benefit in 1967. Annemarie Dührssen, for example, also played a major role in this. The process of professionalization continued.

The characteristics of a profession as distinct from an occupation lie, in addition to academic training and scientifically based special knowledge, above all in the autonomy of professional practice, an exclusive authorization to practice the profession and in professional norms (codes of ethics, collegial-corporative self-regulation). (cf. Geissler, 2013).

These ethical codes have developed and differentiated in the professional discussion. The Freudian rule of abstinence was not without controversy and was variously understood or given content. This process was in its infancy during the period in which the professional discussion of boundary violations in psychotherapy flared up, in the late 1980s and 1990s. And there were still no legal means of action against psychotherapists who violated boundaries.

Irmgard Vogt summarized the (usual) consequences for the perpetrators at the time in the hearing of 1991 as follows: "Although almost no one forgets the information or notification that a colleague has had or is having an affair with a client, most people shy away from sanctions. (...) Mostly it remains a completely non-binding conversation about 'the affair', which does not lead to any consequences. (...) In this way, colleagues become confidants who try to protect themselves against their own knowledge by remaining silent and looking the other way" (Vogt, 1991, p. 68f.).

And these confidants were not exceptions. In 1987 Gartrell, Herman and Olarte had interviewed 1423 psychiatrists in the USA. 65% of them knew of colleagues who had sexual relations with patients. None of them intervened. Most of them regarded these contacts as harmless. For the authors, this finding was the occasion for an urgent appeal to pay more attention to training (quoted from Bossi, 1994, p. 54).

However, Becker-Fischer and Fischer do not see a solution in stricter admission procedures or changed training courses. Rather, they advocate for improved education of the entire profession of therapists, sensitization for borderline behavior, regulated procedural rules in the event of knowledge of abuse among colleagues, and a change in attitude, particularly with regard to the credibility of patient statements in this area (Becker-Fischer & Fischer, 2018, p. 48).

This relegates the quality control of therapy, but also of training, exclusively to the internal world of the institutes or associations. In the sense of a classical profession, it is about mechanisms of self-education, self-control and self-judgement through professional association sanctions for violations of self-defined principles and rules. This reference to the classical profession of the medical profession was obvious, after the profession of psychotherapists had leaned more and more on the medical model, not least because of the approval by the health insurance companies.

> *The answer to the question of how psychoanalysts have responded to burning and pressing contemporary problems is as follows for the post-World War II period: They reorganized their recruitment modalities and selection criteria, thereby changing the specific sociological composition (sample) of their members; they upgraded their institutions so that they became capable of imparting specialized knowledge, isolating them from the rest of the human sciences, and preventing social action potentials; and they used medicalization to overcome their status as an insubordinately critical fringe group and to connect with a powerful, integrated, and conformist stratum of the service sector.* (Parin, 1978, p. 392).

Parin diagnoses a development here that coincides with a pragmatic attitude of post-war psychoanalysis, such as that taught in the Berlin AOK Institute. This attitude – according to Parin – prevented, among other things, participation in social discourse, but perhaps also a self-critical examination of intra-professional developments.

This form of professionalization also leads to the fact that external control of professional action is avoided as far as possible. The profession controls itself. As a side effect, it is very difficult for patients to find a point of contact in the case of treatment errors and boundary violations that takes care of the patient's side. This is still the case today.

Victimizations

The consequences of boundary violations for the affected patients were finally discussed publicly in the 1990s. Committed psychotherapists stepped out of the confines of professional self-control. Books on the subject appeared, newspaper and magazine articles were published. According to Heyne (1991), the consequences of boundary violations and abuse of power range from shock and confusion, not wanting to acknowledge the abuse, trivialization, distrust of others and of one's own self and inability to relate, to psychosomatic reactions, severe depression, abuse of addictive substances and/or suicidal tendencies.

The term "patient sex syndrome" was coined for this in the American literature (Bossi, 1994, p. 64).

According to Becker-Fischer and Fischer, it is irrelevant whether sexual intercourse had occurred, whether sexual touching had occurred, or whether hidden sexualizations had taken place (Becker-Fischer & Fischer, 2018, p. 84f.).

Contact Points for Victims

In the 1990s, there were hardly any contact or counselling centers for affectedpatients. Although the network of counselling centres for women and children affected by sexual violence developed further in the 1990s, women affected by domestic and/or family violence were the main focus. Institutional violence was taken up, affected children were included in the focus, but the topic of boundary violations in psychotherapy led a shadowy existence.

The debate about boundary violations in psychotherapies and the various empirical studies on this led to an awareness also in the various psychotherapeutic training institutes and associations. At the end of the 1990s, a network of committed therapists emerged, which finally led to the foundation of the association "Ethics in Psychotherapy", or "Ethics Association" for short, in 2004.

Although affected patients were able to take legal action from 1998 onwards, it soon became clear that this path was too much for many of them and that they needed support and advice throughout the process. The founders of the Ethics Association began to offer counselling, to accompany patients through the legal process and to support them in their search for follow-up therapies. In the meantime, a collegial exchange takes place in the form of conferences and workshops; the consultations are also documented and statistically evaluated.

Since 2004, more than 1500 consultations have been conducted, including more than 500 in 2017–2019.

Another anchor is the association meetings against boundary violations and sexual abuse in psychotherapy and psychosocial counselling, which have played and continue to play a major role in ensuring that ethical guidelines have been put into effect in the various associations and that the topic of boundary violations has found its way into training and further education.

For the affected patients there is the possibility to file a criminal complaint and/or to sue for compensation for pain and suffering or damages under civil law. It is also possible to file a complaint with the health insurance company, the chamber of physicians or psychotherapists or the respective professional association. However, all of these ways have a multitude of prerequisits and are not made easy for the affected patients. For many, finding the channels of complaint alone is too much, especially since they are usually insecure and vulnerable.

Although various complaint channels and contact points can be found on the Internet, the Ethics Association is usually mentioned in the first place. It works on a voluntary basis and has few human and material resources to support the estimated 300–600 victims per year in Germany.

Thus, the demand of committed experts that there must be more independent and publicly financed contact points for psychotherapy patients remains. There is also a lack of independent patient counselling for therapy patients, especially since the UPD (Independent Patient Counselling Germany) was taken over by a private company in 2016. Since then, the independence of the counselling has been questioned from various sides. Specialized counselling for psychotherapy patients has no longer been offered since 2016. Hurt patients need an independent and professional, low-threshold counselling option that can also accompany them through the proceedings. Information on this can be found on the website of therapie.de (n.d.).

"On the one hand, it is important to stabilize and strengthen the ego functions of the hurt people through low-threshold counselling and support, and on the other hand, through more expert jurisdiction, to contribute to criminal proceedings losing the deterrent and re-traumatising quality for victims that we have unfortunately observed in some of the – in any case extremely rare – proceedings" (Schleu et al., 2018, p. 19). The ethics experts therefore plead for better networking between lawyers and psychotherapists.

Some 30 years after the beginning of a more intensive discourse on boundary violations in psychotherapeutic relationships, there is still much to be done.

7 System Dynamics

The procedure described in the methods section for evaluating the various data sources led to the formation of various categories with explanatory value.[1] According to the idea of grounded theory, based on dialectical movements of thought between data analysis, contextual information and theoretical considerations, an overarching category can ultimately emerge in many research fields, which in a sense provides a hermeneutic framework for many, if not all, of the fundamental findings of an investigation (cf. Glaser and Strauss 1998, 2009; Jaeggi et al. 2004). In the course of our study, it was finally possible to identify such a meaningful explanatory frame, which provides a fundamental contribution to the understanding of the handling of the "Causa H. M." at AKJP-Heidelberg (see Fig. 7.1).

This basic dynamic can be described as a tense dialectic between a functional pragmatism of the system "training institute" on the one hand and the threat to this functional mode by the discussion of sexual transgressions within its own ranks on the other. From this perspective, it becomes clear that failures to perceive, uncover and deal with sexual violence were an integral part of the "normal" functioning of the institution. Seen in this light, all indications pointing to or reminding of the problem of sexual violence represented disruptions of regular everyday processes. Against this background, ignorance, trivialization and rationalization appear not only as strategies of personal defence against guilt and responsibility, but also as functional modes of a superficially successful organizational development.

[1] See also the approach of Burka et al. (2019) in a similar study: "Emergent themes were combined into clusters of connected themes" (p. 254).

P. Caspari et al., *At some point there has to be peace and quiet!*,
https://doi.org/10.1007/978-3-658-39785-2_7

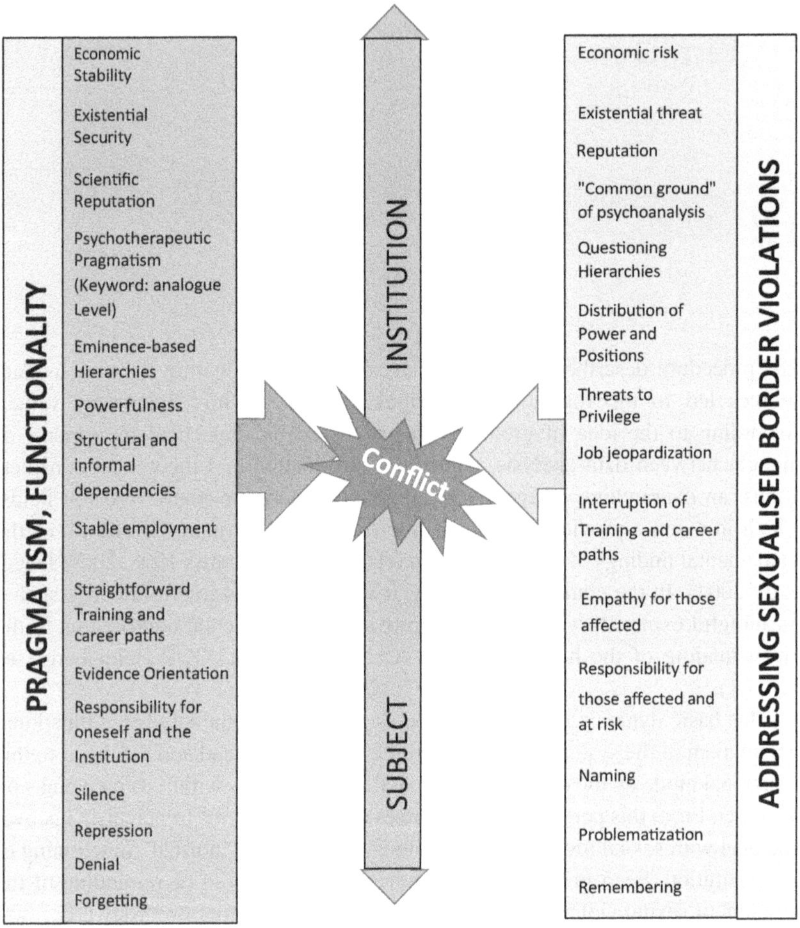

Fig. 7.1 Central basic dynamics of the handling of the "Causa H. M." at the AKJP-Heidelberg. (Own representation)

It can be seen from Fig. 7.1 that numerous and very heterogeneous manifestations, which could be identified from the data collected, can be classified in this basic dynamic. Before these are subjected to a more detailed data-based examination, some preparatory observations are required:

- Aspects of the metadynamics between functional pragmatism on the one hand and the discussion of sexual boundary violations on the other are represented both at the institutional level and at the level of individual subjects. However, depending on the content of these aspects, there are differences in the extent and nature of such representations. For example, the scientific reputation of AKJP-Heidelberg had an identity-forming significance primarily for the institute itself, but only for relatively few individuals employed there. Amnestic defensive processes, in contrast, are also clearly observable at the level of the individuals we interviewed, whereby the figure of an institutional forgetting can also be clearly demonstrated in retrospect. Both academic reputation and the mode of forgetting can be located in the field of tension between functional pragmatism and the discussion of sexual boundary violations.
- The relationship between these two areas is not static by nature. Rather, it can be demonstrated that movements in one area seem to act as triggers for movements in the other. Cover-ups, downplaying or reference to insufficient knowledge of events often represent reactions to threatening attempts at disclosure and thematization because they ostensibly guarantee the functionality of the system. Conversely, the "smooth" functioning of the system can evoke impulses for thematization and scandalization elsewhere because something has not yet been sufficiently dealt with.
- The analogy to a "classic" psychodynamic coping conflict is clear: the unresolved issues from the past irritate the everyday functionality of the individual: conflict, confrontation and discussion trigger anxiety and open up the possibility of coping.
- The concept of functional pragmatism could suggest ethical freedom from contradiction. In fact, however, it has – unsurprisingly from a psychodynamic point of view – a destructive "flip side". Metaphorically, one could also speak here of a Machiavellian "reason of state" that subordinates everything to the "uncomplaining" functioning of the system. The functional pragmatism of AKJP-Heidelberg included, among other things, sexual violence, financial intransparency, serious abstinence violations, structural dilettantism, etc....
- The identified dialectic is crucial from a systems theory perspective because it also directly addresses the question of the existence of the system. At least part of the sometimes overwhelming dynamics of the "Causa H. M." can be explained by the fact that the discussion of his sexual boundary violations can be experienced as an immediate threat to the existence of the institute. The pragmatic functionality of silence results, for example, from the retrospective observation that the exercise of sexual violence by the director of the institute for

18 years was apparently compatible with the existence of the institute without any problems.

These brief remarks lead to a main thesis, which we formulate very simplified at this point on the basis of our research, in order to systematically deconstruct the statements hidden therein in the following chapters with reference to their implications:

In the years 1975–1993 it was reasonable, sensible, pragmatic and functional for weighty reasons to largely ignore all indications of sexual violence by the head of the institute and to refrain from corresponding investigations. It was also sensible, reasonable, pragmatic and functional from 1993 onwards, for weighty reasons, to largely avoid a systematic disclosure of his acts and a sustained investigation into the consequences for the Institute. The fact that the AKJP-Institute Heidelberg still exists gives these "good reasons" a convincing legitimacy. They are the "good reasons" of the institution and the materially secured psychotherapists. But they are opposed to what has not beenworked through and what cannot be put to rest.

7.1 History and Structural Integration of the Institute

In the interviews, in order to understand the background of the Institute and the role of H. M.'s role, the naming of different affiliations to psychoanalytic associations is disguised. Above all, the abbreviations DPG, DPV, and DGPT function as historical and identification-creating localizations of psychoanalytic attitudes and frames of reference.

Due to the specifically German history and the confrontation with the National Socialist past, the conflicts between different psychoanalytic currents were predetermined.

The "Deutsche Psychoanalytische Gesellschaft" (DGP) (German Psychoanalytic Association) emerged from a working group founded by the psychoanalyst Karl Abraham in 1908. Initially, the working group was called "Berliner Psychoanalytische Vereinigung" (BPV) (Berlin Psychoanalytical Union). In 1926 the later name finally emerged. In 1938 the DPG dissolved, but continued to exist as "Working Group A" in the "German Institute for Psychological Research and Psychotherapy", the so-called Göring Institute. The anti-Semitic and totalitarian decrees of the National Socialists led to the exclusion of Jewish analysts in the DPG and to an adaptation of psychoanalysis to the guidelines of a "German Soul Medicine". About 100 analysts and training candidates had to leave Germany because they were Jewish.

In 1945, the DPG was re-established, initially under the name "Berliner Psychoanalytische Gesellschaft" (Berlin Psychoanalytical Association), and from 1950 again as the "Deutsche Psychoanalytische Gesellschaft" (German Psychoanalytical Association). Within the DPG there was a conflict between Harald Schultz-Hencke and Carl Müller-Braunschweig about how to deal with the Nazi past, but also about the admission of non-physician psychotherapists. This conflict led to the resignation of Carl Müller-Braunschweig and a group of analysts from the DPG and to the founding of the "Deutsche Psychoanalytische Vereinigung" (DPV) (German Psychoanalytic Association). Already in the following year, 1951, the DPV was accepted into the International Psychoanalytical Association (IPV).

Both analytic associations are organized in the umbrella organization of the DGPT (Deutsche Gesellschaft für Psychoanalyse, Psychotherapie, Psychosomatik und Tiefenpsychologie) (German Association for Psychoanalysis, Psychotherapy, Psychosomatics and Depth Psychology), which was founded in 1950, partly on the initiative of the American occupation forces. Its first chairman was Viktor von Weizäcker.

The dispute within the DGPT was pre-programmed. The DPG continued to be accused of insufficient distancing from the National Socialists during the Third Reich, which culminated in the founding of the DPV described above. The differences between the respective currents also related to the question of whether psychotherapy should only be practiced by doctors. In addition, different psychoanalytic schools were represented in the various associations (Freud, Jung, neo-analysts). Another conflict arose over the required frequency of teaching-analytic sessions during training and over the question of whether psychotherapy should be conducted exclusively as psychoanalysis. This in turn was followed by different assessments of the competence of psychiatrists in relation to the practice of psychotherapy.

Despite several nascent tendencies towards division, the DGPT has been able to establish itself permanently as an umbrella organization. This is mainly due to the care structure of psychotherapy as a statutory health insurance benefit. Lockot (2010) quotes the DGPT chairwoman Ina Weigelt (term of office: 1981–1983): "When it came to money, the conflicts stopped" (p. 1234).

The AOK Institute in Berlin, which was close to the DPG, played a major role in the implementation of psychoanalysis as a health insurance benefit. The director of the institute, Annemarie Dührssen, presented a study as early as 1962 that provided evidence of the effectiveness of depth psychologically based psychotherapy and psychoanalysis (Dührssen 1962; Dührssen and Jorswieck 1965). This study was the basis for the recognition of guideline psychotherapy as a standard care service of the health insurance funds. The AOK Institute was founded in 1946 as a direct successor to the Berliner Zentralinstitut für Psychogene Erkrankungen (Berlin Central Institute for Psychogenic Diseases), later the Institut für Psychogene Erkrankungen der Allgemeinen Ortskrankenkasse (Institute for Psychogenic Diseases of the Berlin General Local Health Insurance Fund), and was still called the "Göring Institute" for a long time. The original director was Harald Schultz-Hencke.

The AKJP-Heidelberg was founded in 1952 by Annemarie Sänger and was always close to the Berlin Institute of Annemarie Dührssen. In the course of these connections, H. M. also came to Heidelberg in 1975, after Annemarie Sänger had brought the institute into a difficult professional and financial situation. H. M. was to ensure the rebuilding of stable structures. The conditions found at AKJP-Heidelberg seemed to give him a free hand in this respect. In the double role of doctor and analyst all doors were open to him to build up a system in which certain dependencies could be created (for more details see below).

The adult institute IPP-Heidelberg-Mannheim (Institut für Psychoanalyse und Psychotherapie Heidelberg-Mannheim e. V.) (Institute for Psychoanalysis and Psychotherapy Heidleberg-Mannheim e.V.) was founded in 1969 under the umbrella of the DGPT. An assignment to DPG or DPV was deliberately avoided, as can be seen from the following quotation from a key person we interviewed:

"That was important in that it wasn't an institute of one association, so it wasn't DPV or DPG, it was deliberately a mixed institute."

7.2 The AKJP Institute Heidelberg as an Economically, Scientifically and Therapeutically Oriented System

The website of AKJP-Heidelberg states that the institute "has a long tradition dating back to the post-war period".[2] This statement also contains information about the persistence of an organization that has obviously managed to continue a certain psychotherapeutic and institutional line of tradition over many decades to the present day, despite considerable crises. Regardless of the professional or even personal position one may take towards AKJP-Heidelberg, the fact of a basically successful development must be acknowledged, which has led to the permanent establishment of the Institute as a stable psychotherapeutic institution.

These observations refer to the aspect of securing the existence of the organization, which is usually implicit but very significant for our analysis. We can also speak here in the Luhmannian sense of a system defined by the affiliation of certain

[2] See at https://www.akjp-hd.de/das-institut/historie/

positions and elements and the absence of everything that does not belong to the system (Luhmann 1994). This system was endangered in its existence at least twice in the course of history, whereby it becomes clear that precisely these existential threats provide important explanations for the way the AKJP-Heidelberg system dealt with the "Causa H. M.".

First of all, the question of what H. M. contributed to securing the existence of this system is of interest here. The corresponding "founding narrative" places H. M. in the vicinity of a "saviour" after Annemarie Sänger was no longer available as director of the institute she had founded from 1973 onwards. According to reports, the existence of this institution, which was already rich in tradition at the time, was seriously in question. Improvised interim solutions were found, with Karl Tornow taking over the institute's management and the institute secretary Mrs. B. taking on impotant tasks. However, the existence of the institute was not reliably secured until H. M. took over the management. The doctor, who had been brought from Berlin mainly at the instigation of the head of child and adolescent psychiatry, M. P., evidently proved quite quickly to be very capable and suitable for consolidating the existence of AKJP-Heidelberg. This "success story" is of eminent importance, since H. M.'s contribution was not simply to fill a "good job", but his work had an existential dimension for the system he led from the very beginning. As a doctor, he made an important contribution to the economic stability of the institute, since the billing of psychotherapies for children and adolescents within the framework of health insurance benefits formally required a medical director of the institute. In addition to his reported ability as a capable organizer, his excellent networking in the Heidelberg psychotherapy scene also contributed to H. M.'s ability to lead the Institute into a phase of unchallenged existence. The frequently cited "Berlin networks", which refer back to the AOK Institute and Annemarie Dührssen and which are associated with prominent names in the Berlin and Heidelberg psychotherapy scene, proved to be highly functional for the stabilization of AKJP-Heidelberg. From the point of view of securing its existence, these networks proved to be very helpful and profitable for the "Children's Institute". As an adult psychotherapist, H. M. was also organized in the DPG, which enabled him – and thus ultimately also the AKJP-Institut Heidelberg – to make further important professional connections. Regardless of the question of the professional or theoretical reputation of the "child therapy" developed by Sänger and continued in its tradition by H. M. in the eyes of adult psychotherapists, H. M. was able to establish the "Children's Institute" in the Heidelberg psychotherapy scene at least to the extent that there was no doubt about its fundamental right to exist. It was also helpful that he initiated personnel-structural connections by having highly respected medical adult psychotherapists take up certain – more or less formal – positions (as board members, members of the scientific advisory board, lecturers or supervisors) at the Children's Institute. However, the fact that there were also limits to these network formations is indicated in the following quotation from a representative of the adult institute IPP-Heidelberg-Mannheim:

> *Yes, the DPG school, the very conformist school that was completely alien to us, to our generation. So they've never been able to connect properly either, and yet they've had a lot of power. And M. P. brought H. M. here, and there was always a connection. H. M. was then also, because he is also an adult analyst, was also a member of our institute.*

From this overview it becomes clear that the question of existence is of crucial importance when one tries to fathom the dynamics in connection with the accusations against H. M. related to sexual violence. It becomes clear why the defence against these allegations was intuitively and at times explicitly linked to the question of the continued existence of the Institute. In view of H. M.'s "undoubted" merits, the persuasiveness of a discourse figure becomes comprehensible, according to which it was not the sexual boundary violations of the director that endangered the existence of the institute, but the persistent attempt to expose these boundary violations.

Through increased cooperation between the AKJP-Heidelberg and the Heidelberg University Hospital, another existential dimension takes on increasing importance, namely the scientific foundation of psychotherapeutic work with children and adolescents at the Heidelberg Children's Institute. This dimension is not only significant for reasons of reputation, but it was also important in the context of the emerging psychotherapy reform towards the end of the 1990s and the definition of guideline procedures associated with it, which would find recognition as health insurance benefits. The AKJP-Heidelberg, like all other training institutes, had to "position" itself in order to meet the further training requirements associated with the psychotherapy guidelines and to be able to survive on the "market". What was to be feared here was a possible crisis of legitimacy for analytic child and adolescent psychotherapy, since it suffered overall from a lack of empirical evidence of effectiveness.

The efforts of a group of executives at the AKJP-Heidelberg, who wanted to generate empirical data within the framework of a research cooperation with the University Hospital Heidelberg, aimed at remedying exactly this problem, which should contribute to an improved scientific justifiability of the psychotherapeutic procedure at the AKJP-Heidelberg (and of analytical child and adolescent psychotherapy as a whole) (Fahrig et al. 1996).

In addition, a psychotherapist interviewed by us:

And, of course, it is also extremely important from a professional political point of view, because psychoanalysis, psychoanalytic theory ..., therapy was increasingly being attacked and also increasingly questioned, and studies were enormously important; and thus politically, but also important in the community and gained in reputation, because people said that without it we would soon be out of the window. So. And then they started and did big studies; and J. S. supported him very much with his know-how. And those were important things.

The evaluation paradigm, which was primarily based on quantitative data in the context of this research, did not remain free of contradictions in the psychoanalytic scene, since the logic of the psychoanalytic method cannot per se be depicted with the help of standardized measurement models. Regardless of this, a number of important publications on analytic child and adolescent psychotherapy resulted from this research cooperation in the course of the 1990s and 2000s, for which some members, managers and employees of AKJP-Heidelberg were jointly responsible (Fahrig et al. 1996; Horn et al. 2005; Kronmüller et al. 2005; Winkelmann et al. 2000). Therefore, it is permissible to state that the AKJP-Heidelberg has made relevant contributions to the scientific foundation of analytical child and adolescent psychotherapy in Germany.

For the present context, these scientific activities are to be classified in the described "existential paradigm", since they contributed not insignificantly to the continued existence of the Institute after the disclosure crisis in 1993 and established a certain reputation of the AKJP-Heidelberg in the professional public. The research activities realized within the framework of the cooperation with the Heidelberg University Hospital are thus clearly recognizable as a strategy of functional pragmatism of the AKJP-Institut Heidelberg, which saw itself threatened by the disclosure of H. M.'s sexual boundary violations. An unmistakable indication of this is the personnel composition of that group which drove the research activities at AKJP-Heidelberg. H. M. himself, as a good organizer and networker, had contributed significantly to the success of the cooperation with the Heidelberg University Hospital. The fact that his friend and former companion in Berlin, J. S., was appointed director of the Psychosomatic University Hospital in Heidelberg in 1989 was certainly also conducive to this cooperation.

The project of the empirical foundation of analytic child and adolescent psychotherapy and the establishment of the AKJP-Heidelberg as a "science-affine" training institute thus stood on reliable legs. The fact that this existentially important segment of organization and identity continued to exist after H. M.'s departure, or even developed further in a recognizable way, was due above all to A. A., who attached great importance to scientific research and committed herself accordingly in this area.

It is symptomatic that some of the people who particularly pushed this renowned area of the scientific foundation of the psychotherapeutic work at the AKJP Institute Heidelberg also emerged as the people who more or less actively blocked attempts to uncover H. M.'s sexual boundary violations. This makes two things clear: firstly, that the scientific cooperation represented the functional pragmatism of the institute, which by its very nature could not be reconciled with an in-depth examination of the accusations against the head of the institute. And secondly, that this superficial pragmatism at the same time also contained personal and emotional entanglements which had to be fended off together with the accusations against H. M.: The sexual relationship between H. M. and A. A.. The private entanglementof A.A. with the young woman of H. M.. The later love affair between J. S. and A. A. The male friendship between J. S. and H. M.. All this is played out behind the façade of strict, objective, standardized scientificity and the soberly reasoned foundation of analytic child and adolescent psychotherapy. All this seems to contribute to the fact that the protagonists' view of the real accusations against H. M. is obscured. There was a threat at any time and in the long term of the collapse of professional and personal authority based on exclusive hegemonic knowledge. Here it becomes particularly clear how fundamentally the maintenance of the functionality of the institution is entangled with the functionality of the subject.

The ambition to prove the effectiveness of the psychoanalytic process with the help of an inferentially statistically oriented evaluation methodology also presupposes a certain basic understanding of psychoanalysis. The group around J. S., H. M. and A. A. assumed that what is going on in psychoanalytic psychotherapy can be mapped with the help of parameters that would allow proof of effectiveness, of efficiency, in the form of change measurements. Such an approach can be justified in terms of scientific theory and forms the basis for a large part of German-language psychotherapy research, but it also starts from premises that are quite challenging and not entirely uncontroversial. It refers to manualizable disorders within the framework of a medical understanding of illness and health, the symptoms of which are to be alleviated or cured by therapy. This scientific logic, which is only sketched out here, has a high persuasive power: it is reasonable and pragmatic and primarily obeys a cost-benefit paradigm. But it also presupposes a certain understanding of psychoanalysis. It thus assumes a psychoanalysis that can be operationalized within the framework of statistically determinable measures of difference and effect sizes.

This fits with the information we have received about the professional orientation of AKJP-Heidelberg in the era of H. M. – and also afterwards:

But this method did, because that was very anti-analytical, as I see it, pragmatic, purposeful, toward social adjustment, this whole group.

Most of our interviewees expressed satisfaction on the whole with what they had learned at the AKJP-Institut Heidelberg. Apparently, they were not dealing with a dogmatic, orthodox understanding of psychoanalysis, but with a basic orientation that can be described as eclectic. Within the circle of lecturers, different analytical schools and attitudes were represented, so that one could get to know a broad spectrum of therapeutic approaches. Nevertheless, this professional "arbitrariness" was not uncontroversial, especially among those who represented a Freudian-based basic understanding of psychoanalysis in the sense of a "common ground". From the perspective of adult psychoanalysis, the therapy taught and practiced at AKJP-Heidelberg was sometimes smiled at, especially since for a long time it was still considered to be close to the old "psychagogy" represented by Dührssen and Sänger. The suspicion that the therapeutic orientation prevailing at AKJP-Heidelberg was not a "real" psychoanalysis was reinforced by various positions taken by the director of the institute. He propagated a "sober", pragmatic form of child and adolescent psychotherapy with the so-called analogue level. Two related aspects can be described as symptomatic in the present context: First, H. M.'s unusual and provocative professional positioning, which consisted of even casting doubt on the existence of the Oedipus complex, and thus childlike libidinous desire. This was commented on by one interviewee as follows: "Well, the idea of him that these tendencies do not exist at all was completely contradicted by the fact that he acted out and lived out these tendencies completely".

And secondly, the therapeutic refrain from transforming the symbolic enactments in the child's play into the level of linguistic representation. One interviewee sees a connection here to the not coincidental mode of imposed silence, which is typical of sexual abuse: "And I think in retrospect he has – it suits him, of course things should not come up that urgently need to be brought up".

In a similar vein, Burka et al. (2019) remark on the importance of language precisely in the context of managing serious institutional crises: "Under the best circumstances, at the symbolic level, words and symbols themselves are able to function as 'containing objects'. But when symbolic thinking is constricted, language can be confused or corrupted" (p. 265).

On a metaphorical level, the basic pattern that is at the center of the present discussions emerges here again: Functional pragmatism on the one hand, rejection of verbal discussion on the other. With the denial of the Oedipal conflict, desire is banished from the world of the child. It seems as if the child's libidinous desire is the phantasm of unteachable psychoanalysts, but in the sober, pragmatic, symptom-oriented therapy world of H. M., J. S. and A. A. such empirically elusive phenomena have no useful place. In this concretist world, freed from phantasms, the doctor takes very real hold of the penises of little boys. This world is also content with playful acting on the analogous level; in this world the joker H. M. appears at institute parties, as a childlike prankster and enchanting actor. This world is obviously not only "sober"; rather, its pragmatism also unites the playful, the foolish and the perverse. What it completely lacks, however, is the reflexive-analytical penetration of real events and their symbolic representations on a verbal level. Therefore, the discussion of the sexual boundary violations perpetrated by H. M. appears as the most threatening attack on this world in which playful acting out in child psychotherapy is so dependent on an inferentially statistically based scientific legitimation. The production of "objective data" thus not only had the function of enabling the AKJP-Heidelberg to establish itself permanently, both scientifically and economically, but it also served as a "blessing" of a certain understanding of psychoanalytic work with children and adolescents, which was by no means perceived without contradictions. At this point it should be recalled once again that this elaborate and demanding scientific alibi was produced and propagated, among others, by those persons who most actively blocked the efforts to clarify H. M.'s sexual boundary violations. From the point of view of a representative of the IPP-Heidelberg-Mannheim, this connection is not coincidental:

> *It's that school. They don't think about reappraisal. They think pragmatically. We have to look to the future, reach our goal. It's simple.*

The dialectic between the functional maintenance of the existence of the AKJP Institute Heidelberg on the one hand and the endangerment of its existence through the discussion of the sexual violence perpetrated by the Institute's director H. M. on the other hand was finally manifested again in a concise manner through the court proceedings against H. M. and the appearance of the article in the "ZEIT" (Aisslinger and Lebert 2018). The tense debates in connection with and in the wake of these two events pointed to the enduring character of this dialectic, which was also recognizably incorporated into the commissioning of the scientific inquiry of sexualviolence.

In fact, 25 years after H. M.'s resignation, the question of the Institute's existence was once again raised, when the discussion of the events of that time in a broad public was at stake.[3] One person from the Institute's environment expresses these concerns succinctly: "My worst fear would be that the Institute is finished, also financially and in terms of its name".

In a symptomatic way, the fronts between functional pragmatism and persistent scandalization hardened almost "inevitably". The central argumentation figures of those who advocated pragmatic positions with a view to an undisturbed, reliable "course of operations" were primarily the following: "We have enough tasks that require our attention and energy. Why should we dwell on old, long-gone stories?", "Publicly dealing with the sexual violence perpetrated by the former director of the institute and not adequately stopped by the institute damages the reputation of the institute.", "A large-scale scientific investigation costs a lot of money and therefore endangers the financial stability of the institute." It is apparent at first glance that these arguments have a persuasive force based on reason. To refute them requires a great deal of argumentative effort and exposes those who insist on a publicly visible investigation of the case to the suspicion that they are exposing the Institute's existence to incalculable risks. This dialectic continued during the research process, especially in that phase when it was a matter of preparing public appeals in the media – with the aim of finding victims who had suffered sexual violence at the hands of H. M. in the past. Damage to the institute's reputation and the threat to its existence came to the fore as fundamental threat scenarios and had to be weighed against the demands of an investigation that is also dependent on the voices of the victims.

At the end of these remarks, two insights seem central to us: As long as attempts to (publicly) address H. M.'s crimes at the AKJP Institute in Heidelberg lead to a reactance that appeals to the maintenance of the Institute's existence, its good reputation, its scientific reputation and functioning "operating procedures", there seems to be a dynamic that makes it necessary to work through the past. And: It requires at least a thorough reflection on the fact that functional pragmatism, as legitimate as it may seem, has proven to be a rather poor advisor in dealing with the "Causa H. M." over a long period of time. The economic and reputational question

[3] Cf. similar fears in Burka et al. (2019) in connection with the publication of an article on the inquiry of serious ethical misconduct at their own institute: "We recognize that anxiety is an inescapable factor in any discussion or presentation that spotlights ethical violations, so this article may generate anxieties" (p. 261). And even more clearly: "In order to engage in writing the article, we had to examine our fears that we too could be participating in wrongdoing by breaking the code of silence. The question of publication inevitably exposes the tension between containment and transparency. Attempts to contain can be experienced as keeping secrets and colluding against transparency. Attempts at transparency can be seen as overexposure and violations of confidentiality" (p. 262).

of existence is "of course" central for an organization. But its seductive power lies in the defense against problematic developments and dynamics that such an organization makes possible and allows under its ostensibly functioning umbrella (cf. also the "negative example" of the Odenwald School), which ultimately had to file for insolvency and cease to exist in the wake of the exposure of the systematic sexual violence perpetrated there (Keupp et al. 2019).

7.3 Professional Identity/Organizational Identity

The institutional dynamics described in the previous section find relevant equivalents at the subject level. In the following, it will be shown that questions of existential and economic security as well as professional reputation and identity make an important contribution to the question of why, for a long time, no systematic and sustainable attempts were initiated in the environment of the AKJP Institute Heidelberg and at the institute itself to uncover and end the sexual boundary violations of the institute's director. Corresponding effective dynamics can be proven on three levels, namely on that of the training candidates, the employees and the responsible persons at the institute.

With regard to training candidates, it should first be pointed out that learning the profession of psychotherapist was and is associated with both an extraordinarily high time commitment and a considerable financial outlay. Those who decide to take such a step accept significant changes in their own lifestyle for many years. Everyday life is grouped around seminars, treatment cases, supervisions, interventions, teaching analyses, whereby it is not only about learning professional skills, but especially in psychoanalytic training it is about a profound, intensive, long-lasting examination of one's own person. Those who choose such training are making a life decision. According to our interviews, the corresponding motivations are the desire for professional change, personal development and ultimately also stable financial and existential security. Many of those we interviewed did not see any permanently satisfying career prospects for themselves as teachers or social pedagogues and therefore considered the possibility of qualifying as a psychotherapist as an attractive life perspective. In some cases, the founding of a family was seen as a reason to ensure one's own livelihood in the long term with the help of psychotherapy training. The prospect of eventually no longer simply being employed as a teacher, social pedagogue or psychologist, but of having one's own practice as a child and adolescent psychotherapist was not only associated with financial incentives, but also with a significantly enhanced personal reputation. The training at the AKJP Institute Heidelberg was therefore a central identity project for the majority of the candidates, which made it necessary to stay "on track" for many years, i.e. to meet the diverse training requirements that strongly affected the individual.

In view of this explanation, it becomes clear how necessary and useful the acquisition of a functional pragmatism was also on the individual level of the training candidates working on their professional careers. The high expenditure of time and money had to "pay off" after all. In addition, something else is important. The close link between professional qualification and personal involvement, which is characteristic of psychoanalytic training, allows questions of identity work to emerge not only in connection with the formal fulfilment of training requirements and the structurally secured achievement of professional goals in the form of a branch. Aspects of identity also configure themselves from the affiliation to particular therapeutic schools or currents, to professional associations, and not least to a particular institute in which one's own professional and psychotherapeutic socialization was substantially shaped. Professional identities are as important as they are fragile. They play a significant role in the reassurance of one's own self and one's own actions. Against this background, it does not seem to require further explanation that damage to the reputation of the institute at which one was trained is quite inevitably associated with damage to the reputation of one's own professional persona (Slochower 2017). All training candidates and all subsequent psychotherapists therefore have a fundamental interest in having been trained at a 'good' institute, one that is highly regarded in professional circles and, more importantly, one that lays the foundation for developing confidence in the quality of one's psychotherapeutic practice (Burka 2008; Wallace 2007). At this point, an important function of defending against evidence of the institute director's crimes becomes apparent: the potential scandal at the institute can lead to the cessation of teaching and the interruption or even termination of training. But the problem remains virulent even in retrospective observation: having been trained at the "H. M." Institute means that one's own professional socialization took place in a milieu marked by the sexual boundary violations of the director and by the more or less silent complicity of his collegial environment. In our interviews we encounter – with a few concise exceptions – defensive tendencies in this regard: There had been nothing wrong with the quality of the training. Regardless of the misconduct of the head of the institute, one could qualify as a capable child and adolescent psychotherapist. One did not have much contact with the head of the institute anyway; there were a number of very experienced lecturers from whom one could learn a lot. The special professional work of A. A. was emphasized in many places, from which many training candidates benefited. The professional reputation of H. M. himself is also evaluated positively by contemporaries. He had been "a good diagnostician", had had unconventional ideas for treatment, etc. It seems that one's own professional identity was and is experienced as largely untroubled by this training milieu contaminated with sexual boundary violations and abuse of power. Only occasionally do former training candidates ask fundamental questions about their own professional identity, either because they have always had reservations about the professional orientation of the institute or because they are horrified by the abysses that are gradually opening up in relation to the AKJP Institute Heidelberg.

The conscious and active confrontation with the sexual boundary violations of the head of the institute involved and still involves considerable risks for the training candidates at the time: Factual endangerment of the costly, demanding and elaborate training path and: Questioning of their own professional identity as practicing child and adolescent psychotherapists, because the unmasking of the "H. M." Institute as a system of abuse would be associated with a reinterpretation of their own professional narrative, which would be linked to a critical perspective on their own actions and on themselves as psychotherapists. In this context, Burka et al. (2019) speak of a "moral we" by which a psychoanalytic institute is latently held together and which is fundamentally challenged by ethical (e.g. sexual) misconduct of an authoritative person. The collective unconscious of a group of trainees and colleagues is deeply irritated by the recognition of the fact that the ethical principles of psychotherapeutic work have been turned into their opposite. No one who belongs to the psychotherapy institute can escape this shock, because "this is a version of me as a member in this group" (p. 263). Since the individual unconscious is entangled with the collective unconscious of the group, individual identity issues are inexorably forced upon the group when the group structure is shaken by the sexual transgressions of a significant member.

In view of these remarks, it seems all the more remarkable that in 1993, when the first accusations against H. M. were made, a small group of training candidates formed, who actively campaigned for disclosure of the sexual boundary violations and for H. M.'s immediate resignation. These individuals were concerned about "their" institute in a different way than anyone else involved. They saw the danger of isolation or dissolution of the institute in the event that its abusive leader was not immediately and uncompromisingly gotten rid of. They were self-critical of their failure to be diligent in not noticing the evidence of sexual boundary violations and not taking steps towards stopping them. They expressed this as co-signatories of a corresponding letter of the regional group of the VAKJP. In the research interview, these persons still raise questions decades later about the damage to their own professional identity by the events at AKJP-Heidelberg. Despite the risks involved, they left the path of functional pragmatism at that time and entered into a fierce conflict dynamic within the institute. They were largely isolated with their attitude within AKJP-Heidelberg and did not receive any support from the adult institute either. They had to struggle with powerful currents that were oriented towards the pragmatic preservation of threatened identities (cf. Burka et al. 2019).

What was described above in connection with most training candidates is probably even more valid for former employees and managers. This is true in several respects, but there is also a serious identity dimension involved. The answer to the question of whether one could do high-quality psychotherapeutic work in an institution whose director sexually exploited children and adolescents as well as young female patients, training candidates and colleagues cannot be answered without contradiction from the outset. The reference according to which one "didn't have that much to do with the institute and its director" is symptomatic against this background. The safeguarding of one's own professional identity happens through what one has not done and not experienced. The connection with the AKJP-Heidelberg and with its director, once recognized as a professional authority, is assigned a marginal position in the perception of one's own professional socialization. In this context, at least two temporal phases and different degrees of involvement in the AKJP-Heidelberg system are to be distinguished.

The first phase, which spans the years 1975 to 1993 and in which H. M. was apparently able to commit sexual boundary violations against various groups of people relatively unchallenged, appears in retrospect to be unobjectionable for employees and responsible persons in terms of identity. This is especially true with the help of the discourse figure that one knew nothing of the deeds of the head of the institute. The second phase is more complicated, since the indications of these boundary violations brought to the institute from outside make a positioning necessary. At this point it becomes apparent how strongly the mode of functional pragmatism comes into play in those people who feel connected to the AKJP Institute Heidelberg: the hints are dismissed, because there is a lot at stake: securing one's own job, one's own professional position, securing one's own reputation and thus: Defending one's professional identity. These fundamental processes prevented a real and sustainable "reinvention" of the institute as long as representatives of the "old system" continued to hold decisive positions. One of their strongest motives for action was to defend their own professional and personal identity, created over many years with a great deal of effort and commitment, at all costs. The fact of reciprocal influence had a particularly lasting effect: Not only was the professional identity of these individuals decisively shaped by the AKJP-Institute Heidelberg, but they themselves also influenced the organizational identity of AKJP-Heidelberg in leading functions in the further course. Some of these persons were actually identified with the institute and continued to shape the professional orientation, the structures, the interpersonal interaction and the atmosphere of the institute, which could sometimes appear like this to new training candidates:

> *Small-minded. Maybe by narcissistic needs, boundaries, small-minded, small-minded, by – yeah, maybe by all these prohibitions on thinking, prohibitions on speaking, vulnerabilities, bigotries, that kind of climate blew up on me.*

It is important to understand that part of this identity consisted of "not letting the accusations against H. M. become too big", because a comprehensive disclosure and inquiry would have massively called into question one's own overall biographical project and the functionality of the institute that was closely linked to this project. It was all the more important in this phase that "good work" continued to be done and that "operations" were kept running as undisturbed as possible.

In this context, it is also important to observe that many former training candidates turned away from "this institute" because they no longer wanted to have anything to do with a certain type of organizational identity that had been decisively shaped by the long-established staff and responsible persons. Some terminated their membership in the supporting association, others let it rest and refrained from further involvement in association matters. All this does not exclude that from the mid-1990s onwards there were staff members at the Institute who were not identified with the old "H. M. Institute", but who had professional and personal connections and networks beyond the complex of AKJP-Heidelberg, University Hospital and Child and Adolescent Psychiatry. For these persons it was not an immediate threat to their professional identity to name the grievances in connection with the "Causa H. M.", since their professional and personal self-assurance was not so strongly dependent on an undamaged image of the AKJP-Heidelberg.

This also applied to those persons who had a high reputation in the Heidelberg psychotherapy scene and who were connected with AKJP-Heidelberg for various reasons (e.g. because of personal relations to H. M. or because of their interest in the therapy of children and adolescents). These were the medical colleagues M. P., J. S. and M. K., who held high positions in clinics or at the adult institute and at the same time acted as members of the board or the scientific advisory board of AKJP-Heidelberg. In addition, some of them held lectureships at the Children's Institute. Their role is interesting because their professional identity was by far not as strongly linked to the AKJP-Institut Heidelberg as was the case with those staff and board members who worked exclusively as child and adolescent psychotherapists and were also institutionally primarily bound to the AKJP-Heidelberg. The medical colleagues referred to here, on the other hand, had much more important professional, financial, specialist and network-related footholds outside the AKJP-Institut Heidelberg. Their high reputation was nourished by their work in the clinic sector and in the field of adult psychotherapy. It can therefore be stated first of all that neither in the case of M. P. nor in the case of J. S. does the "identity argument" have sufficient explanatory power for their refusal to make an effort to consistently clarify the accusations against H. M. They could have retreated to the position that they did not have too much to do with the Institute anyway and that no one "would have lost their face" of their high professional reputation if they had clearly distanced themselves from H. M. and taken a clear position with regard to his deeds. The opposite, however, was the case: M. P. as well as J. S. and M. K. continued to be committed to the AKJP-Institut Heidelberg, namely by taking over the function of the provisional head of the institute, by filling a position on the board and by continuing a research cooperation on a permanent basis. In this way, they supported in a fundamental way those forces at the Institute who had inseparably linked their existence as well as their professional and personal identity to an AKJP-Heidelberg constructed as impeccable. These highly respected medical colleagues, by virtue of their authority, functioned as elementarily important protective shields for the old forces at the Institute, whose identity depended to no small extent on the cover-up of H. M.'s deeds. Symptomatic in this context is the role of M. P., who took over the leadership of an institute about which he had often made rather disrespectful comments. As a psychoanalytic professor of medicine, he simply did not take seriously the psychotherapy practiced at AKJP-Heidelberg and the psychotherapists responsible for carrying out the therapies. To take over the management of an institute for whose working methods and staff he had above all contempt left, is an initiative that definitely needs explanation. At least it becomes clear here that the prominent gentlemen were not concerned with identity issues when they placed themselves protectively before H. M. But they flanked the identities of the established AKJP-Heidelberg employees who saw themselves so massively threatened by the accusations against H. M. Superficially, all three men mentioned here made significant contributions to the maintenance of the Institute's existence: one took over the provisional leadership at a time of the highest crisis (which is strikingly reminiscent of H. M.'s "rescue" in 1975), another took over responsibility as a board member and later led the inquiry group, and the third established a permanent research cooperation and thus contributed significantly to the Institute's reputation and economic stability. These are therefore prototypical representatives of functional pragmatism, which secured the existence of the Institute and also the professional identity of the "old guard" at AKJP-Heidelberg. If one is involved in an abuse system in this way, one simultaneously takes a certain position towards the sexual violence perpetrated within this system. That means: In these cases, too, a commitment to the clarification of the acts would not have been compatible with the functional pragmatism that served to maintain the AKJP-Heidelberg system. In favour of the three persons mentioned here, however, it can be stated that at that time the institute could not be identified as a system of abuse. The "misconduct" of a single individual, which could not be proven in a justiciable way, no concrete accusations by parents or caregivers, no known statements by affected students of teaching analysis or training candidates. The visible result of sexual exploitation – having children with the patient – seemed to be "legalized" by the marriage. H. M. s behavior was sanctioned insofar as he felt compelled to relinquish his leadership position. Seen in this light, contours of an abuse system only become discernible from a temporal and analytical distance.

Since the identities of M. P., J. S. and M. K. were not connected to the AKJP-Institute Heidelberg, other reasons probably contributed to the fact that they did not clearly position themselves against H. M. and for an explanation of his deeds. It can be assumed that these reasons, at least in the case of M. P. and J. S., were mainly of a personal nature. As respected physicians and psychoanalysts, they had "mingled themselves" with a colleague whose personal deficits were already recognizable at an early stage and whose professional ethical missteps had been known for a long time. It is simply embarrassing not only to work professionally with "someone like that" but also to be personal friends with him. It fulfils a self-identity-protecting function if I don't let the extent of my friend's depravity become too great, since in all this there is also information about my own social and emotional judgement. Surely such a capacity should be presumed in psychotherapeutically trained clinic directors. The fact that all three of them lack the ability to judge the dynamics of sexual violence is an additional explanatory factor, which is also not consistent with their professional competences.

From the perspective of identity theory, it becomes clear why AKJP-Heidelberg rotated in a peculiar-seeming field of tension between concealment on the one hand and attempts at disclosure on the other in the decades after the allegations against H. M. became public. There were highly relevant and powerfully supported couplings between a personal and professional identity and an organizational identity. Even when L. Z. took over the leadership of the institute in 1994, AKJP-Heidelberg continued to be shaped in a decisive way by forces that did not sufficiently distance themselves from the professional orientations, the structures and the atmospheres of the old H. M. Institute:

> *Let's put it this way, you'd have to look a little more closely: Who was on the board at that time? And who had (...) the say in the institute, let's say. Right? Or what were the leading figures? Or something like that. Maybe you could look at it a bit more that way. I think that has a lot to do with A. A., that there was no impetus that might have promoted us: Continue there. Right? Or we have to uncover that or something. But of course there was always a brake in it, right? That's what I would say.*

For these old forces, the initiatives of clarification brought in from outside, and in the meantime also pushed within the Institute, continued to pose a fundamental threat to their professional and personal identity. Therefore, the disputes in this regard almost inevitably took the form of "existential struggles", which were associated with a correspondingly pronounced emotionality.

7.4 Power, Dependencies

In the previous explanations it was shown in which way institutional as well as individual self-interests contributed to the concealment of the sexual violence carried out by H. M. at the AKJP-Heidelberg. These self-interests were described as "reasonable", legitimate and pragmatic, because they primarily aimed at a consolidated reputation, economic stability and a recognized professional identity.

We have spoken above – rather metaphorically – of a kind of "Machiavellian reason of state", with which the context of justification of these self-interests can be sketched. The events surrounding the "Causa H. M." cannot be adequately understood if the technique that helped such interests to break through is not subjected to a closer examination. Here, by way of introduction, the convincing finding must be reported that the organization of interests took place within a framework that was characterized in a decisive way by a serious inequality in the distribution of power. Symptomatic of this is an immediately striking, almost absurd abundance of power, which H. M. had at his disposal during his entire time as head of the AKJP Institute in Heidelberg: "Well, he was the board of directors, chairman, everything in one person, teaching analyst, he put his own people on the couch there, completely crazy. So that was a mixture of functions without control."

Power and its reciprocal dependence function as central explanatory figures in the analysis of the events surrounding H. M. Power is a basic condition, concomitant and stabilizer of all forms of sexual violence that H. M. perpetrated against different groups of people. In order to do justice to the heterogeneity of relevant aspects of power, a bullet point list of corresponding constellations is provided here:

- The "initiation" of H. M. at the AKJP-Heidelberg in 1975 was associated with an anticipatory feeling of gratitude on the part of all those involved. They were prepared to transfer far-reaching competences to him, so that he would be able to lead the institute, which was endangered in its existence, into a stable future.
- H. M. acts at the AKJP-Heidelberg as head of the institute and chairman of the association's board in personal union. He also managed the finances of the

institute. For a long time, this allowed him a largely non-transparent financial conduct, which only towards the end of his activity increasingly triggered questions and irritations among individual members of the association.

- As a doctor he was at the top of the informal as well as formal professional hierarchy of AKJP-Heidelberg. He used the "prestige difference" between training candidates, employees and himself, which consisted in the fact that people who were "only" trained as teachers, social pedagogues or psychologists "looked up to" him as a medical doctor. This professional inequality was further reinforced by his position as a delegated doctor, since the performance of any psychotherapy at the institute required his approval.
- H. M. had powerful friends at his disposal, most of whom resulted from his professional socialization in Berlin and his affiliation with the DPG. He was close friends with, among others, the head of child and adolescent psychiatry and with the later head of the psychosomatic university clinic in Heidelberg. M. P., the head of child and adolescent psychiatry, had brought his friend H. M. to Heidelberg so that he would take over the direction of the children's institute. His work at the adult institute IPP-Heidelberg-Mannheim gave H. M. an additional boost in reputation as an adult therapist and educator of adult psychotherapists.
- By bringing his physician friends and colleagues from the clinics and the adult institute to the AKJP-Heidelberg (where they occupied various positions and acted as lecturers), H. M. cemented his already seemingly limitless power at the AKJP-Heidelberg.
- Within the framework of the training at the AKJP-Heidelberg, H. M. acted as lecturer, supervisor, second examiner and examiner. Whether he carried out teaching analyses at the AKJP-Heidelberg cannot be established beyond doubt in retrospect. However, it is undisputed that due to the functions he fulfilled, all training candidates were in a partially extremely pronounced relationship of dependence to H. M. The same can be said about his role at the adult institute IPP-Heidelberg-Mannheim, where he at times chaired the selection committee and the examination board.
- Assessment and therapeutic situations with children were characterized by a blatant imbalance of power, which was not limited by any control mechanisms. The sexual exploitation of the children was perpetrated by H. M. in his functions as an adult, as a man, as a doctor, as the head of the institute, as a delegating authority, as a scientist and professional authority.
- What is valid for the therapeutic situation with children is also valid for the therapeutic situation with adolescents. In addition to other aspects, the power available to him to shame his patients also comes to the fore here.

- When committing sexual violence against young adult female patients, H. M. also resorted to the apparently unrestricted power that the psychotherapeutic setting gave him. In this way he was able to make use of a rich spectrum of manipulation possibilities, which paved the way for sexual exploitation.
- For the sexual exploitation of supervisees, training analysands and other candidates for training, H. M. made use of the a priori existing relationship of dependence to which the women were subjected. This was characterized by one of the experts interviewed by us as follows:

> "The [psychoanalysis trainees, author's note] are even in a double dependency, because they also want to finish their training, they can't defend themselves at all. Besides, they have to open up."

- With A. A. H. M. placed a person in a leading position at AKJP-Heidelberg who was entangled in a dependent relationship with him in many ways. She had completed her training at AKJP-Heidelberg and was protected and promoted by H. M. as a capable child and adolescent psychotherapist, organizer and theoretician. A. A.'s professional identity was thus particularly closely linked to AKJP-Heidelberg. She first worked as a lecturer and later became chairman of the board at AKJP-Heidelberg. That she was involved in a sexual relationship with H. M. is clear from his diaries. After H. M.'s resignation she continued to represent his interests at AKJP-Heidelberg.
- A. A. is a particularly prototypical example of a more general pattern of granting or refusing emotional attention to training candidates by the head of the institute. H. M. had his "darlings" with whom he surrounded himself and who, under his wing, decisively shaped the culture and atmosphere at AKJP-Heidelberg.
- The emotional attention granted by the head of the institute was not infrequently linked to concrete privileges that H. M. granted to individual trainee candidates. Such informal favours formed the basis for a system of loyalties and dependencies that H. M. practised for years and with which he secured his position. By not being so particular about admission requirements, by generously acknowledging training components that had not been completed, by advocating the approval of training graduates who did not actually fulfil the relevant requirements and by showing understanding in the case of longer interruptions of training courses, he not only acquired the gratitude and loyalty of those privileged in this way, but also created effective dependency relationships, i.e.: he had it in his hands to cause serious problems for the training candidates if they did not behave loyally towards him.

- His relationships with the young female patients with whom he had children in common were also marked by a serious imbalance of power and dependence. There is no doubt that he involved his wife E. M. in a system of abuse that was sustained not only by emotional but also, and in particular, by a blatant degree of economic dependence. The joint children, the lack of a professional perspective, persistent psychological problems and living in H. M. s house constituted obstacles for E. M. which could hardly be overcome for a separation from the wealthy doctor and psychotherapist with whom she had sought help for her psychological burdens as a young woman. The relationship with R. R., the mother of his son, was also marked by dependencies. It is possible that R. R. succeeded in escaping emotional dependence. However, we only have diary statements by H. M. on this. Through their common son, however, a lifelong involvement with H. M. persisted, which also consisted of joint drug consumption and loose sexual contacts.
- After his resignation from the AKJP Institute in Heidelberg and his resignation from the DPG, H. M. obviously still had functioning networks that protected him from the withdrawal of his expert activities and his function as an expert advisor for psychotherapy at the health insurance company.
- When allegations were repeatedly made against H. M., he used the extremely effective means of power of threatening libel charges with the help of his lawyer. In an aggressive manner he made use of the silence of the victims in order to put the informers in the vicinity of perpetrators who would move on the edge of breaking the law with their allegations.
- H. M. countered any accusations of sexual transgressions against child patients (which led to at least two criminal investigations against him) with recourse to his professional authority as a medical doctor who had the power to proclaim diagnostic requirements as he saw fit.

This list requires a systematization. This refers first to the contexts and then to the way in which power is exercised.

7.5 Contexts of Abuse of Power

Essentially, three areas can be distinguished from each other, within which H. M. established his specifically designed power regimes. It is evident that these areas mutually affect each other in many ways and thus altogether connect to a very stable power complex.

Psychotherapeutic setting: This first area is at the centre of the events that are the subject of the present investigation. It forms the stage for the majority of those scenes in which H. M. perpetrated sexual violence against boys, girls, adolescents, adult female patients and trainees. The scene of the psychotherapeutic setting is thus transformed into a crime scene, and it is important to understand that fundamental structural conditions are present here that favor the abuse of power and the sexualization of interpersonal interactions (Becker-Fischer and Fischer 1996; Hirsch 2012; Schleu et al. 2018). Two aspects in particular can be identified that are crucial for corresponding risks: Hermetic isolation of the situation and asymmetry of the relationship. The primary risk dynamic is that this asymmetry is associated with a manufactured inequality of power potentials and that the abuse of such a constellation is promoted by the exclusive, hermetic character of the setting. This is a fundamental problematic of the psychotherapeutic setting that must be constructively translated through precise framing, abstinence bids, and a commitment to a consciously reflective approach to the manufactured asymmetry (Hirsch 2012). H. M. s behaviour is a glaring reminder of the risks involved in producing such a setting. It is therefore all the more remarkable that, when asked whether the field of psychotherapy/psychoanalysis is particularly vulnerable to possible boundary violations, we frequently received responses in our interviews that corresponded to the following statement by a psychotherapist: "Nah, I don't think so; no more vulnerable than anywhere else."

H. M. realized that the exclusive, asymmetrical encounter gave him a degree of power that, by analogy with the "total institution" (Goffman 1973), was based on impenetrable boundaries on the outside and a complete lack of boundaries on the inside (Caspari, forthcoming; Enders 2002). In view of the assessment that H. M. was not a pedosexual offender, it can be assumed that it was not so much sexual needs that drove him to his acts, but rather the special constellation of the psychotherapeutic setting that opened up an area of unrestricted power for him. The "savoring" of this power was achieved with the help of the genitalization, eroticization, sexualization of the situation: touching boys by the penis, asking questions about masturbation practices, grabbing adolescent girls by the breasts and asking them about their sexual experiences, engaging young female patients in erotic play, transferring the teaching analysis into the realm of private relationships, etc. All of these practices have a common origin, a common motive: gaining pleasure through an excess of power made available to the doctor and psychotherapist through the exclusivity of the hermetically organized psychotherapeutic setting. Or more pointedly, he does it because he can. It is clear what the asymmetries are in each case: The child doesn't know whether it's usually necessary to take off one's clothes when making an indication for psychotherapy. The young person cannot assess whether shameful questions about sexuality might not be part of "normal psychotherapy" after all. The young patient feels flattered by the extraordinary interest that the doctor takes in her "of all people". The same is true for supervisees, training analysands and staff members who have been chosen for a special form of intimacy with the highly respected institute director, doctor and psychotherapist. A psychotherapist interviewed by us:

> *Well, he did have a sense of what was going on with the other person. You have to hand it to him, he abused that, yes, but he had that. And he really always picked – either those who were weaker, or he picked those who wanted to participate narcissistically.*

The potential for abuse of power and manipulation appears inexhaustible, with some evidence suggesting that H. M. was quite interested in the extent of the spectrum of this inexhaustibility.

In the present context, the particular resistance to disclosure of the psychotherapeutic setting is also important. Everything that makes the disclosure of sexual violence difficult appears here in compressed form: Ambiguity of the event, boundless shame, guilt reversal, manipulative power of the perpetrator, lack of verifiability of the event. Or as one interview partner puts it:

"Well, there was a time when you didn't believe a patient because he was a patient. Today it's more like you believe everything because he's a patient."

The following recent experiences of a psychotherapist (cf. also Schleu et al. 2018) show that this assessment by no means contributes to the fact that disclosures of sexual boundary violations committed in the context of psychotherapies would be easier for the victims in the meantime:

> *So in the last few years I have of course often been approached, by the way always via supervision, and have always encouraged patients to contact an ethics officer, for example. And although these patients know that the ethics officers do not automatically take action and file any charges, I can only remember one case out of five or six where a patient even took the opportunity to speak to a person. So that's where the reverse gear is put back in incredibly quickly.*

The multifaceted arrangement of obstacles to disclosure is based on the power of those who use the psychotherapeutic setting for narcissistic enhancement, psychological violence and sexual exploitation.

AKJP Institute Heidelberg The children's institute run by H. M. constitutes the second sphere of power which he made use of in the perpetration and cover-up of sexual violence. We have seen that at AKJP-Heidelberg he set up informal and formal structures which enabled him to control the institute almost in a way analogous to that described above for the psychotherapeutic setting. As head of the institute, as chairman of the board, and as delegation doctor, he held all the positions that allowed him an unrestricted power regime that seems astonishing in retrospect.[4] Therefore, it did not cause him too much difficulty to group this regime around those psychotherapeutic settings in which he committed sexual boundary violations. It is important to note here that the technique of exercising power was not ostensibly authoritarian. Rather, it was organized in a cooperative, one might even say manipulative, manner. All trainees and employees more or less got along with the director of the institute. Some kept their distance, some did not like him very much, others, however, tended to move in a close circle around the head of the institute, one or two colleagues went to bed with him. As far as we know, all of them were able to achieve their educational and professional goals in their own way, without overtly suffering from the structurally invested power of the institute director. The forms of informal exercise of power seemed to have had rather positive connotations for those concerned. One was not harassed, marginalized or devalued by H. M. in an extraordinary way, as is reported in individual cases in connection with the era of M. P. Informal exercise of power was expressed by H. M. rather in the granting of the above-mentioned favours (e.g. recognition of training requirements not fulfilled etc.). A "small favour" could sometimes consist of drinking a glass of wine with the supervisor H. M. after the supervision and imagining oneself as a member of the circle of his "favourites". Such favours created dependencies and their structural context was always a pronounced asymmetry of power. The eroticization of interactions, the sexual experience, and the years of sexual relations with extended travels always had their origin in the constellation of power described here.

An example of the consolidation of such constellations was the conspicuous maneuver to get a lecturer position at the AKJP-Heidelberg for a teaching analyst from the adult institute with whom H. M. had had a sexual relationship for years. A. A.'s career at the Children's Institute must also be seen against this background: She was brought into her positions by the director of the institute, H. M., from which she decisively influenced the fate of the institute for decades. Her original

[4] Krutzenbichler's (1998) characterization of the position of power of psychotherapists is very fitting: "Someone who, in narcissistic misjudgment, puts himself in the place of the law, embodies it powerfully-institutionally in the sense of the word-cannot be guilty – he is, after all, the law" (p. 323).

socialization at the AKJP-Heidelberg took place exclusively on the basis of H. M.'s regime, which was organized by pronounced power and dependence. Against this background, it is rather unlikely that their joint sexual relationship came about free of these asymmetrical dynamics.

It is important for our context that H. M. s sphere of power at AKJP-Heidelberg was very robust against possible suspicions regarding abstinence violations. The clearest example of this is his handling of the widely known fact that he had had a child with a female patient since 1980. Two aspects are of primary concern here: first, that people were generally satisfied with the information that the young woman had been impregnated by H. M. only after psychotherapy had ended. And secondly, that H. M. himself – and even more so his secretary – revealed this story in no uncertain terms, at least to the public of the institute. The boy who had resulted from this relationship showed up at the AKJP-Institute Heidelberg again and again in the following years, whereby H. M. presented himself as a caring father. This self-assurance staged by the institute director seems brazen in retrospect, but is to be interpreted primarily as a symptom of his unrestricted power at the institute.

H. M. created a milieu at the AKJP-Heidelberg, which was characterized by power relations, which on the one hand seemed quite socially acceptable, but on the other hand also made abstinence violations, seemingly harmless eroticizations and sexual violence possible in an oppressive way. After the disclosure of sexual violence, H. M. had to give up this unrestricted regime. The fact that disclosure and inquiry subsequently proceeded in a fragmented manner at best had to do with the fact that the power relations established by H. M. continued to be effective – at least partially – despite his departure.

Networks The networks of H. M. outlined above, which to a large extent had emerged during his time in Berlin and were able to unfold in Heidelberg in an effective way, formed a further sphere of power which, so to speak, macrosystemically wrapped itself around the asymmetrical scene of the psychotherapeutic setting and the "domain" of the AKJP-Heidelberg. There is nothing to suggest that these networks, consisting of prominent and powerful representatives of the Heidelberg psychotherapy scene, actively contributed to the cover-up of the acts committed by H. M. However, they allowed themselves to be instrumentalized by H. M. in a conspicuous manner in order to secure his position of power, which was necessary for committing and cover-up of sexual violence. Not least by referring to these powerful friends, H. M. was able to establish and consolidate his reputation as a capable doctor, psychotherapist and institute director. He succeeded in this all the more by providing them with certain positions within his sphere of power of the AKJP-Heidelberg structures and/or by entering into cooperations with their clinics.

These networks played a major role especially during the disclosure of the sexual violence and in the following years, when it was important not to let the extent of his crimes become visible and not to endanger his professional foothold as an expert witness, expert advisor at the health insurance company and psychotherapist in private practice. In this context, however, the functioning of these networks remains largely intransparent. However, their effect and the profit of power can be seen in the fact that H. M. was able to continue to work unchallenged for many years and to successfully defend himself, when attempts were repeatedly made, with good reasons, to discredit him at the health insurance companies and in the expert committees, especially on the part of the adult institute IPP-Heidelberg-Mannheim, the VAKJP and finally also the AKJP-Heidelberg.

Above all M. P. and J. S., but also the married couple T. as well as M. K. functioned as pillars of a system consisting of different spheres of power, which enabled H. M. to practice sexual violence without being bothered and permanently protected him from serious consequences. It would have been necessary for these prominent physicians and psychotherapists to expose this function (in the sense of a functionalization or instrumentalization) as such in time and to no longer assert their own power (also in a passive way) to secure the power of their colleague H. M. Even if they distance themselves from their own involvement in the "Causa H. M.", their power was never irrelevant in this story. Using it responsibly on the basis of careful reflections might have contributed to different courses and processes.

7.6 Nature of the Exercise of Power

To better understand how power asymmetries work, it is important not only to illuminate the contexts of H. M. s abuse of power, but also to point out different ways in which power is abused (cf. Helfferich et al. 2021).

Agency As described above, the psychotherapeutic setting provided H. M. with a paradigmatic context that enabled him to commit sexual boundary violations and assaults. He was therefore empowered to act insofar as there was no authority that could have put a stop to him in the concrete situation. He was able to make children undress, he was able to touch young women and he was able to actively eroticize the interaction with training candidates because the psychotherapeutic setting allowed all this from his point of view.

This extent of agency was also available to him within his "domain" at AKJP-Heidelberg. As head of the institute he was able to establish those formal structures and launch those informal manoeuvres that consolidated his position and entangled his staff and trainees in dependencies that were both symptom and support of his regime based on agency.

Interpretive Power The potential inherent in the power of interpretation is an everyday tool of psychoanalysts. The misuse of interpretive power, in turn, is a constitutive element of all sexual violence (Mosser 2020). This justifies the necessity of consciously and reflexively perceiving the corresponding risks inherent in the psychotherapeutic (and in particular the psychoanalytic) setting. The case of H. M. is virtually prototypical for the extraordinarily high importance of the power of interpretation in connection with sexual violence. He made use of the power of interpretation granted to him by his professional position in a variety of ways in order to manipulatively conceal the acts he was able to commit by virtue of his power to act. The fact that this happened in an almost excessive manner and that this extent of interpretative power in particular ensured that the acts were not brought to any critical discussion for such a long time points to the destructive possibilities inherent in psychotherapy. In short: The manipulation of the victims and the manipulation of the environment apparently represented routines of the psychotherapist H. M. that had been practiced for decades. The power to do this was primarily given to him by his professional position. It was easy for him to reinterpret every sexual assault against children and adolescents as medically or psychotherapeutically legitimized action.

The fact that one has to undress at the doctor's or that one has to put up with more precise questions about one's own sexuality in psychotherapy is a kind of *common knowledge* that nips the discomfort about such experiences in the argumentative bud, decisively limits the possibilities of resistance and taints the communication to the outside world with serious doubts. Having to reenact a sexual assault one has suffered, or having a therapist concretely demonstrate how to have sex, are experiences that adolescents may not anticipate in terms of psychotherapy, but which can be reinterpreted by a reputable psychotherapist as "helpful interventions." The very act of shaming ensures silence and thus prevents the potential inclusion of people who might well place other interpretations.

It is clear that the initiation of sexual relations with young adult female patients were also completely subject to the interpretative regime of the psychotherapist: The asymmetry between the woman who had just become an adult and had been socialized in the youth welfare system and the doctor, psychotherapist, and institute director, who was almost 40 years older, is by all means not limited to a difference in agency, but manifests itself to an even greater extent in the differentially available possibilities for interpreting situations, interactions, actions, relationships, and the world at large. This is the prerequisite for enduring and variant manipulations.

Teaching analysis and psychoanalytic supervision present situations that are by definition characterized by interpretation. And they open up the possibility for the teaching analyst and supervisor to use such settings for manipulation and the perpetration of violence through the abuse of the interpretive power ascribed to them qua their position (Burka 2008; Sandler and Godley 2004; Wallace 2007). H. M. made ample use of this possibility. Whatever his interpretive maneuvers may have looked like, they contributed in several cases to an eroticization and sexualization of teaching analyses and supervisions and formed the basis for sometimes long, sexual relationships. Moreover, it must be taken into account here that the cognitive process of interpretation takes place against the background of a specific emotional constellation that is constitutive of psychoanalysis. The therapeutically induced regression of the patient is not least the aspect that centrally justifies the penal sanctioning of sexual interactions in the context of psychotherapies[5] (Schleu et al. 2018).

In the case of H. M., the importance of a pronounced power of interpretation was demonstrably not limited to his contact with the people he sexually exploited. It also manifested itself in an obvious way in his efforts to defend himself against accusations and suspicions that were launched against him from 1992 onwards. All the figures of discourse that he launched from the time that people began to actively and critically discuss acts that had become known were based on his ability to formulate his own interpretations in a largely unassailable way: "I haven't done any teaching analyses at the Adult Institute for a long time. There were three relationships with women that began years after the completion of the respective

[5] Spieß (1998) describes this basic state of affairs as follows: "Power relationship because, by engaging in treatment, we oblige patients to tell us everything, even the most intimate and embarrassing things – combined with the clear agreement that a reaction/response, which would be adequate/desired under "normal" conditions will not come from us. Under "normal" conditions, only crazy people would engage in such an unequal, impossible relationship. Here, then, the abandonment of reason, autonomy, and self-responsibility is implied, presupposed, from the outset!" (p. 339).

teaching analyses. The relationships with the young female patients did not begin until after they had completed psychotherapy. I am going to marry the patient who currently became pregnant by me. I am not to be blamed for anything. These are consistently adult relationships that are no one's business. The accusations made anonymously against me have no basis in fact."

The power of interpretation proves itself in the fact that it is given to someone. H. M. succeeded with the versions he circulated, which were a mixture of lies, distortions and trivializations, in anchoring the assessment among many people – especially at AKJP-Heidelberg – that it was a matter of largely harmless misconduct, which was quite compatible with a continuation of his office as head of the institute. In particular, there was little objection to his continuing to act as second sifter and delegation doctor. The undoubted facts that he had impregnated two young female patients and had had sexual relations with several training analysands could apparently be ignored within the interpretative regime launched by H. M. H. M. showed himself to be remorseful at members' meetings and in the circle of lecturers, but at the same time he presented a version of events which largely exonerated him. Above all, he complained that he had not been heard by those who had made the accusations against him. Not hearing him out, however, meant limiting his interpretive power by making the communications of those women who had been affected by his manipulations and sexual boundary violations the guiding principle of one's own assessment of the facts. Not listening to him also meant: letting the facts speak for themselves: pregnant patients, deeply hurt colleagues.

The extent of the power of interpretation attributed to him helped H. M., even many years after the partial disclosure of his acts, to be able to exercise his professional functions largely undisturbed. Criminal charges for sexual abuse of children and complaints from female colleagues were lost due to his ability, as a doctor and psychotherapist, to twist the incriminated facts in such a way that they had a seemingly absurd persuasiveness in view of the accusations made against him as a whole. In addition, he succeeded for many years in offering therapy or supervision in the role of expert on the subject of sexual abuse in various institutions, including a correctional institution and a housing project for sectarian dropouts.

After H. M. had resigned from his functions at AKJP-Heidelberg, his regime of interpretation continued to live on there. Influential persons, above all A. A., but also to a limited extent M. P. and many others, held the view that the sexual boundary violations of which the former head of the institute was accused were either unimportant or not so bad. This interpretation routine persisted despite multiple challenges at least until the court case against H. M. or until the publication of the "ZEIT" article in 2017 and 2018. It took a court decision in which H. M. was proven to have sexually abused his granddaughter 11 times to finally bring down his interpretation regime that had been effective for decades.

The considerations presented here are of eminent importance for understanding the case. The power of interpretation of the perpetrator is constitutive for sexual violence: "This is normal", "You like it too". There is no doubt that it is important to listen to people who are accused of committing sexual violence. Serious consequences resulting from unjustified accusations must be avoided at all costs. In the case of H. M., however, sufficient facts were available to make the danger of the unjustified accusation obsolete. Although these did not initially justify a criminal investigation, they were clear indications of serious professional and personal misconduct, about which a consensus should have been reached at AKJP-Heidelberg. However, there was already a lack of a fundamental conceptual understanding about what had happened – as can be seen from the statements of an interview partner from the adult institute:

> *Abuse of power, yes, but, yes, that wasn't called violence either, at most seduction or what, that's violence in that case, because of dependence. But the term didn't appear there.*

It should also have been recognized that the problem of the abuse of interpretive power is an eminently psychoanalytical problem, which should have led to fundamental self-questioning at the AKJP Institute Heidelberg and in its environment.

7.7 Organizational Power

One final aspect of power is presented here for the sake of completeness, in order to fully understand the workings of the dynamics from which H. M. benefited. His power was not only nourished by the possibility to use the psychotherapeutic setting for sexual assaults and to reinterpret these acts in his sense. As could be shown, he also succeeded without difficulty in consolidating his interpretive regime by activating many allies, some of them quite influential. A person's organizational power is expressed in this ability to draw supporters to one's own side when necessary. Everything that has been said above about the sphere of power of the AKJP-Institut Heidelberg and especially about H. M.'s networks contributes to the constitution of this organizational power. He was by no means isolated as *persona non grata at* the moment when he was accused of having impregnated female patients and entangled teaching analysands in love relationships. On the contrary, a powerful and numerically large faction of people formed to follow his arguments and at the same time to be outraged by the aggressive influence from the outside (in the shape of the adult institute IPP-Heidelberg-Mannheim) – a widespread dynamic in the aftermath of serious accusations against "prominent" representatives of an institution (cf. e.g. Dehmers 2011; Sandler and Godley 2004). Despite facts to the contrary, this group perpetuated the image of the unjustly vilified, deserving institutional leader. The exercise of organizational power manifests itself in particular in the technique described above of instrumentalising such individuals as have been useful to H. M. in advancing his interests and defending himself from attacks against him and his professional practice. Exercising organizational power then means, for example: Functionalizing a colleague as maid of honor; inviting colleagues and powerful friends to the wedding celebration; publishing joint professional articles; a joint lecture at the Lindau Psychotherapy Days; taking over second sights "in short order"; sending a colleague with a bouquet of flowers to the hospital to the wife who has just given birth. Organizational power also means: permanent influence on what happens in AKJP-Heidelberg via the "governor" A.A.

In summary, it can be said that H. M. exercised power in various ways in different contexts over decades. In his case, it can also be stated that this concentration of power constituted a direct trigger for the exercise of sexual violence, since the abuse of power in sexual form enabled libidinous gain of an addictive nature. Fatally, this concentration of power not only constituted a precondition for the perpetration of sexual violence, but it also guaranteed the cover-up of the same for many years. The effect of this power prevented the realization of necessary steps to remove H. M. from his profession and to prevent further victims even after the partial exposure of the events.

7.8 Victimizations

At the beginning of the fourth chapter we documented more than 30 scenarios describing sexual boundary violations and assaults by H. M. We have pointed out that this enumeration is a sketch of a bright figure, which undoubtedly points to a much larger dark figure. It can therefore be assumed that a large number of boys and girls, of female and male adolescents, of adult female patients and of female trainees were affected by H. M.'s sexual boundary violations.

There are very few victims who have spoken out about these experiences. If they did so, then in a protected, trusting setting, beyond the boundaries of which the corresponding information often did not reach. A total of four people who had suffered sexual violence at the hands of H. M. confided in us researchers. It is clear from the descriptions in Chap. 4 that reliable information about the victims had to be generated from a complex conglomeration of data sources, which can also be understood as an expression of a deeply rooted culture of secrecy and mistrust in the environment of the AKJP-Heidelberg.

This culture can be demonstrated by the numerous failures to disclose, which are also presented in Chap. 4. In this context, it can at least be summed up that

1. a smaller number of children and adolescents communicated to their parents,
2. a few parents disclosed to their psychotherapists or directly to the Institute that H. M. had committed sexual assaults against their children,
3. two parents filed criminal charges against H. M. for sexually abusing their children,
4. about four or five affected female trainee analysts reported sexual violence by H. M. to an executive of the IPP-Heidelberg-Mannheim and
5. at least two young female patients were impregnated by H. M. and this was also known at AKJP-Heidelberg.

Apart from a criminal complaint filed against H. M. only in 2013, all cases listed here were known at the AKJP-Institute Heidelberg at the latest in the second half of the 1990s. In the present context, it is worth highlighting the observation that although this information was used to take more or less unsuccessful action against H. M. and to make needs for inquiry at AKJP-Heidelberg more visible, there was, on the other hand, apparently a pronounced blind spot relating to the needs of the victims.

The discourse about H. M.'s actions was clearly perpetrator-related throughout all phases. There was intensive discussion about how the accusations against him were to be evaluated, what consequences he would have to draw from them, and what these accusations meant for the Institute. Nothing about this is superfluous; but it is precisely at this point that it again becomes clear how functional pragmatism in dealing with sexual acts of violence in one's own ranks is connected with serious fade-outs, as is also shown, for example, in a retrospective balance sheet of a participant in the group "Past – Present – Future":

> *There hasn't been a communiqué, there hasn't been sort of, 'What do we do with this now?' Or what will follow from it?... but simply left it at that, expecting that this would strengthen the Institute as a whole. Yes? It was also a matter of strengthening the inner life of the Institute, so to speak. That was actually the main task.*

The view of the victims was undoubtedly very weak. The former training analysands who had confided in the adult institute were regarded as the victims. There was talk that they were heavily burdened by H. M.'s sexual boundary violations, but this was to serve primarily as an argument against trivializing the abstinence violations in the dispute about the perpetrator. As far as we know, these women had made use of psychotherapies in order to cope with their lastingly stressful experiences with H. M. Nothing more is known. We have no information about the extent to which the IPP-Heidelberg-Mannheim and AKJP-Heidelberg institutes initiated efforts to express sympathy and solidarity with these women or to give them recognition for their courage in disclosing themselves. We do not know of any systematic reflection on how the institutes could have taken care of these women, but the impression is that they were primarily functionalized: While the faction striving for clarification hoped that the women would report to the criminal investigation authorities and/or to the medical association, the opposing side instrumentalized the silence of the the victims with the argument that the accusations only came from anonymous sources and thus offered no basis for further consequences. In the dispute about H. M., the victims were primarily assigned the role of (non-)informants.

Even more obvious were the failures in dealing with R. R. and E. M. While the sexual relationship of the head of the institute with R. R., which led to a pregnancy, met with practically no critical response from the public, in 1992/1993 the relationship with E. M. was the focus of the controversies about the person H. M. Symptomatic here is also an almost exclusive orientation towards the perpetrator: Are the relationship with the (alleged ex-)patient and her pregnancy compatible with the function of the head of the institute? Did he violate abstinence rules and ethical principles? And so on. The situation of the young woman, who had been socialized in youth welfare, had experienced severe sexual traumatization in her past history and had now become pregnant by the institute director in the context of the AKJP Institute Heidelberg, did not seem to interest anyone seriously.

While some colleagues took part in the secrecy of the first pregnancy, they and others acted as witnesses and wedding guests in order to participate in an abstruse production, the purpose of which was to legitimize a relationship that had come about through an obvious abuse of power. A. A., for example, had known the young E. M. for a long time and knew of her biographical burdens. Nothing seemed to trigger the impulse in her to save the young woman from the abusive relationship with H. M., with whom she herself had sexual contacts. As far as is known, the director of the adult institute IPP-Heidelberg-Mannheim had sporadic contact with E. M. in the following period. The young woman described to her the suffering of her marriage, expressed the wish for psychotherapeutic support and was finally referred to colleagues outside the IPP-AKJP-Heidelberg complex.

With regard to the children whose parents confided directly or indirectly in the AKJP-Heidelberg, no initiatives on the part of the Institute are known which could have contributed to the relief of the victims. The reports were merely documented and, at least at times, used as a reason for discussions and disputes at the Institute. At no time did the Institute seriously and systematically consider how it could have actively and carefully approached former patients and their parents – possibly also in cooperation with external agencies – in order to pave the way for a discussion of irritating or damaging experiences and to find and implement forms of recognition of such experiences. Such activities are costly, complicated and by no means risk-free, whereby it must also be taken into account that at the time there were no known institutional models for working through the past.

However, two observations are symptomatic. Firstly, a comprehensive avoidance of an empathic approach to the victims and an equally comprehensive rejection of possible initiatives to identify, contact and engage with the victims can be reconstructed. These failures within AKJP-Heidelberg and IPP-Heidelberg-Mannheim go far beyond the group of those who avoided any confrontation with H. M.'s deeds in the mode of functional pragmatism. Questions about how victims could be found and addressed, how a credible assumption of responsibility by the Institute could be signaled to them, and what concrete support could be made possible for them in the sense of coping and and working through what they had experienced, obviously remained outside the discourse horizon of all those involved.

At this point the members of both institutes, between whom there were otherwise sometimes deep gaps, united in a common attitude of functional pragmatism. In another psychotherapy institute, in which there was an overlap of personnel with the IPP-Heidelberg-Mannheim, the question of actively approaching the victims was at least dealt with, although the result of such considerations ultimately corresponded to that of the institutes that were directly involved, as we know from the following communication from an interview partner: "Well, it was discussed how that could be done. But nothing happened."

Secondly, the extensive omission of the victims is also reflected in our interviews. Rather, we find indications of a partial co-responsibility of the affected adult women, who were themselves probably emotionally and sexually needy; in addition, we find trivializing levelings of the psychotherapeutic situation, in which things are possible that can also happen elsewhere: "… heard so many things from so many people, where it happens everywhere, at the high school graduation and the teacher, in the dentist's office (laughs), so everywhere where two people come together in affective conditions, it can slip in that direction. And that's a lot of responsibility on both of them, of course."

We find codified reproaches against the victims because they did not file charges against H. M. and thus fundamentally weakened all efforts to clarify the situation:

"So you couldn't say anything to people because they didn't agree. So everything remained covered up."

In this context, one's own helplessness is still warded off years later by aggressive projections and guilt reversals.

In other cases we find a choice of words that leaves no doubt about a lack of empathy towards the children affected: "And then – but now don't ask me how – the accusations came up that he had been looking so intensively at the boys during these delegation talks and that he had always, how do I know, lifted his panties somewhere and looked at their willies. So those are the things I learned afterwards."

One still signals respect towards a former colleague who from a certain point on did not allow any children to see H. M. alone, without recognizing the serious omission that this colleague did nothing further to protect other children except her own therapy children from this therapist. Almost nowhere does the sympathetic question arise as to how these children and adolescents must have fared who were defencelessly subjected to the assessment and therapy situations with H. M. Almost nowhere is the question raised about the victims, of whom one has no knowledge at the Institute and possibly also outside the Institute, and who were faced with the biographical task of having to cope with the irritating, disturbing or deeply hurtful experiences with the doctor and psychotherapist presumably all by themselves. We hardly find a contextualization of the "voluntary sexual relations between adults" into a structure of power asymmetry between the institute director/supervisor/teaching analyst on the one hand and the women dependent on him on the other:

> *That was not in my interest, I was more of the opinion that adult women have to know who they are getting involved with. So from an analytical point of view, of course, one could have absolutely questioned it. But it didn't affect me personally, because I saw them as responsible for themselves, yes.*

This incomplete list of quotations from our interviews with psychotherapists is by no means to be understood as a moral indictment, especially since the attitudes outlined here cannot be generalized to all interview partners. Rather, these positions function as part of an explanatory pattern that is intended to describe the institutional handling of the psychotherapy institutes involved with the actions of the institute director. This pattern is not unusual. The media's treatment of sexual violence is also characterized by a pronounced fixation on the perpetrator. The scandal is ignited by the perpetrator, and the way in which the perpetrator is dealt with proves much more succinctly how institutional action is judged than the complicated and difficult-to-operationalize approach to the victims.

The insufficient emotional involvement with those affected serves as a negative frame for the functional pragmatism of the institution.[6] This mode finds a particularly clear expression in the strategy that could be called "evidence orientation". The lack of evidence is the alibi of the perpetrator and his confidants. The corresponding argumentation figure, which was represented at the forefront and with a high degree of persuasiveness, especially by A.A., was: If the victims do not come out of the closet and if they do not press charges, then our hands are tied. Our task is then merely to make sure that we can indeed do nothing if the victims do not go the way of reporting to the prosecution authorities and to the health insurance companies. This means that if nothing has been proven, there is no need for any consequences:

> *So what I know from A.A. is that her statement was, 'I can't take action unless somebody files a report.' Unless someone reports him, I can't act upon it.*

This reasoning is both understandable and superficially reasonable (even if psychoanalysis is not exactly known for delegating problems and conflicts exclusively to the realm of criminal law[7]). But in the present case it unfolded a powerful effect as a means of power and above all relieved those responsible of the demanding task of opening up ways of dialogue, confidence-building and support for the victims. It was clear that the victims would not turn to A. A. in confidence – this alone represents an oath of revelation for the AKJP Institute Heidelberg. The evidence orientation, as reasonable as it may appear at first glance, functioned in the present

[6] Burka et al. (2019) make a clear connection here to the need for institutional and individual livelihood security described above. The "survival mode" of those involved offers no room for empathy for the victims: "When survival of the group feels at stake, the group may resort to defensive manoeuvres that it would not exhibit in more stable times, such as increased efforts at control, intolerance of difference, and lack of empathy for others" (p. 263). Elsewhere it is described how imposed or perceived institutional silences corrupt the very task of psychotherapists, namely the support of distressed people: "If group anxieties are not addressed or symbolized – due to silencing surrounding the investigation – the shared group assumption of providing care to those who suffer is neglected" (p. 264).

[7] Pfannschmidt (1998), for example, summarizes the discussion about sexual abuse in psychotherapy in the following words: "In my impression, the discussion about remedies polarizes into two irreconcilable positions: On the one hand, there is a plea for adherence to abstinence, which is seen in renunciation and refusal of substitute gratifications. One advocates the introduction of new penal norms because, given the high rate of sexual abstinence violations, this really seems to be the only way to get a grip on the problem; a proposal that is difficult to reconcile with psychoanalysis. The other side tends to the opinion that one should not exaggerate after all (…)" (p. 365).

case as an effective means of power, which permanently muzzled the victims who were struggling for recognition and support.

In retrospect, the impression arises that all initiatives to clarify and come to terms with H. M.'s sexual boundary violations were primarily oriented towards the perpetrator and the organization and less towards protecting possible further victims from H. M. Symptomatic of this is the fact that the concern and indignation of those involved was based much more on his work as an expert than on the fact that he treated children, adolescents and adults in his psychotherapeutic practice in Seckach on a daily basis. This focus seems in need of explanation, especially since it was very persistent and still shows up in our interviews. From an external perspective, it can be said that H. M. did no "immediate harm" with his expert activities – except that one could be outraged by his unchallenged power to decide on the approval of psychotherapy applications. Much more alarming, however, is the fact that he continued to conduct psychotherapies and to act as a second examiner for colleagues who were aware of the accusations against him.

These descriptions are not meant to suggest that it would have been even remotely easy or promising to prevent further patient contacts by H. M. after 1993 (Molitor 1998). However, after 1995, when he opened his practice in Seckach, there were increasing indications at the AKJP-Heidelberg that he committed sexual boundary violations against children in the context of examination situations. According to the information available to us, however, the focus of the initiatives against H. M. continued to be on challenging his work as an expert. However, the goal of all efforts should have been to obtain the revocation of his medical license, since he was known to use the medical-psychotherapeutic profession to commit sexual assaults against various groups of patients. The reference to the fact that nothing corresponding could be obtained if the victims did not file a complaint could at least have released systematic search movements in connection with the question of who the victims actually were: Mrs. E. M., to whom he was married? The former teaching analysts who had their psychotherapeutic practices in the meantime? Or a number of children and their parents who had registered at the AKJP-Heidelberg or with psychotherapists in the second half of the 1990s? We are not aware that the Adult Institute IPP-Heidelberg-Mannheim, the Children's Institute AKJP-Heidelberg, the Youth Welfare Office and possibly the criminal prosecution authorities would have developed strategies as part of a concerted approach that would have had the potential to prevent further victims.

In a certain sense, it seems futile to reproach the protagonists of the time with such subsequent criticism; in the present context, however, these failures appear at least as a symptom of a lack of orientation towards the victims. We do not have any information about how many boys, girls, adolescents and adults suffered sexual boundary violations by H. M. in the period between 1995 and the ultimate withdrawal of his license at the end of 2013. However, it would be very surprising from what we know if he had suddenly refrained from this behaviour, which was identified as addictive, especially as he was still demonstrably committing multiple acts of sexual abuse against his granddaughter in 2016.

At this point the circle to functional pragmatism closes. The identification of victims is complex and complicated; the institutional assumption of responsibility towards victims is emotionally demanding; success in actively approaching victims based on empathetic dialogue is difficult to achieve and requires reflective attitudes and patient work; the prevention of further victims is a goal that is as rewarding as it is difficult to achieve – but the prospects of success in this regard remain mostly speculative, unless the accused is behind bars for a few years – in short: Personal involvement in an institutionally supported victim orientation is strenuous, costly and carries the potential for considerable frustration. Orientation towards the victims – both in its coping-related and in its preventive orientation – requires considerable resources, emotional and professional commitment, reliable cooperation, process-oriented work and a high tolerance for frustration.

Against this background, it seems reasonable and pragmatic to limit one's own activities to complaining to the expert panels and the health insurance companies when once again an expert opinion signed by H. M. flutters into one's house and when one is outraged by the information officially confirmed by the in-house counsel that no one can be removed from circulation if there are no victims who would be willing to testify against him. Repeated discouragements by criminal charges that were not pursued further, by pragmatic legal assessments and by panels of experts who stood behind their colleague H. M., led to an at least partially resigned mode of dealing with the "Causa H. M.", which, however, was disturbed by intermittently newly burgeoning information that reminded one that there was still something wrong here.

It is not the genuine task of a psychotherapy institute to clarify sexual boundary violations in a way that prevents the suspect from continuing to practice his profession. For this there were and are instances with which it is the duty of the respective institute to cooperate (umbrella organizations, chambers, ethics association, youth welfare offices, specialist counselling centres). A large number of these bodies were involved in the case over the years, but in retrospect the picture appears to be one of rampant helplessness caused by fragmentation rather than that of a process-oriented, reliably coordinated approach.[8] In such a constellation it seems inevitable that the psychotherapy institutes actually and mainly turned back to their genuine tasks and impotently accepted the daily dangers emanating from the former institute director: "So we were perhaps also cowardly, yes? Perhaps we were also afraid. I would say so, yes. And as it is, you don't want to have to deal with this shit all the time, do you?"

7.9 Forms of Defence

The following remarks initially refer primarily to the subject level, although a closer look reveals that individual modes of reaction and processing are also reflected at the level of institutional action or omission (cf. Burka et al. 2019; Sandler and Godley 2004; Slochower 2017). These are decidedly psychological processes that are, so to speak, part of the elementary theoretical inventory of psychoanalysis. Nevertheless, these explanations do not claim to have a systematic psychoanalytic foundation. Rather, with reference to our interview data in particular, it should be made clear how "all too human" dynamics also unfold their effect at a psychotherapy institute when psychodynamically trained and working people are confronted with unpleasant things that prompt their own psychological apparatus to seemingly attractive defensive reactions.

7.9.1 Defence of Responsibility

The defense against responsibility is least describable in terms of a psychodynamically justifiable reaction. It can be explained on the surface of human behavior, so to speak. Nevertheless, it will be subjected to a more detailed analysis at this point, because it represents a very concise type of defense that can be determined from our data, which acts as a kind of link between the explanations in the previous sections and the more unconscious defense mechanisms presented below.

All that has been said about institutional and personal pragmatism and a lack of stakeholder orientation can be translated into an argumentation figure that centres

[8] "The board of the Association of Analytical Child and Adolescent Therapists had become very involved in the matter in the interest and on behalf of affected colleagues and had painfully experienced the limits and impotence of honorary court sanction possibilities. The findings from this case speak in favour of demanding criminal and professional regulations for sexual abuse in therapy" (Molitor 1998, p. 332).

on a certain mode of responsibility organization. This becomes immediately understandable if one contrasts three objectives of individual responsibility: Responsibility for oneself, responsibility for the institution, responsibility for those affected and those at risk.

It was worked out that for most of the actors in the context of the "Causa H. M." the focus on affected and endangered minors and adults was rather weak. This was mainly justified by the subjective decision for a functional pragmatism, which suggested a turn towards a task orientation that corresponded to the genuine requirements of a psychotherapy institute. On the other hand, turning to those affected or endangered appeared to be unpromising, time-consuming, energy-sapping, and thus frustrating. In this mode, which could be presented as reasonable, something continued for decades, which was already clearly recognizable during the time in which H. M. still led the AKJP-Heidelberg: The discussion of the question whether persons could be harmed or endangered by H. M.'s activities remained conspicuously underrepresented throughout.

Characteristic of this is the argumentation figure "These are adults. They'll know what they're doing." By virtue of its objective indubitability, this sentence has a high persuasive power and thus acts as a template for the defence against one's own responsibility for the well-being of female colleagues and fellow students. Whether one leaves one's own apartment to a married fellow student so that she can meet there with the head of the institute; whether one sees a teaching analysand leave the house in which H. M. lives in the early morning; whether one accepts a patient's communication in psychotherapy that "H. M. sleeps with his female patients" – all of this can ultimately be transferred, despite considerable inner disquiet, into the assessment that those involved are, after all, adults and that one also has inhibitions about inquiring too closely. It is not so much a matter of taking a moral position as of assessing that an assumption of responsibility for those possibly affected could prove to be highly complex at the level of action. What would an assumption of responsibility consist of for the fellow student in love who wants to spend a few nice days with the head of the institute?

Other questions arise when a psychotherapist receives a second-sight record in which "strange" examination practices of the head of the institute are described. Here the assumption of responsibility for the child victim and for all the children who would still be examined by H. M. seemed to fail due to the assessment that such examination methods are probably medically indicated and thus legitimate. Nevertheless, the rejection of responsibility from an ethical point of view seems to be more serious here, which also explains why such second-sight records only found their way into the arena of discourse of the AKJP Institute Heidelberg with a delay of decades. As such examination records were readable at least for the secretary and the respective treating psychotherapists, H. M.'s practices were known. However, there is no interviewee who told us about a personal confrontation with such irritating protocols. Functional pragmatism then means: The delegating doctor and head of the institute approved my application to carry out psychotherapy, i.e. assumption of responsibility for myself and my professional activity; rejection of my responsibility for the child who was examined by H. M. in a possibly questionable way. The solution to ethical problems could then be to be personally present at the examinations of one's own therapy children, to inwardly assure oneself that one's own therapy children had not been touched by H. M., or to tell parents that they should rather present their children elsewhere. All this leads to the conviction that taking responsibility for myself is in any case more conclusive, less costly and more promising than taking responsibility for therapy children who may not have been harmed anyway or for such children whom I do not know at all and who will be presented to H. M. at some point.

A picture is emerging in which the assumption of responsibility for potentially affected or endangered persons is in clear competition with coping with one's own life demands. Or as Burka et al. (2019) put it, "The 'survival task' may be at odds with the 'work task'" (p. 264). Again and again, we hear of training candidates, staff and managers being heavily occupied by professional and private demands (e.g. because they started a family during the training period and thus lived in a financially strained situation), so that in most cases "more obvious" options for taking on responsibility presented themselves here: responsibility for one's own family, for one's own children, for one's own professional development, for financial stabilization, etc. The most convincing argument for rejecting responsibility is not knowing, as expressed in the following quote from a leader: "I've always wondered why they've been talking for years about something I've never heard."

As long as the rumours about H. M. did not reach the level of a public discourse of scandalization, the defence of responsibility towards affected or endangered persons seemed to be subjectively justified relatively easily. This changed with new forms of contextualization, which became virulent with the partial revelations in 1992/1993: As it was pronounced that H. M. had committed abstinence violations and sexual assaults from which victims suffered, previously valid patterns of appeasement were endangered. However, the defences of accepting responsibility for the victims and at risk were largely maintained. This becomes particularly clear in connection with E. M., around whose wedding with H. M. a larger delegation from the AKJP-Institute Heidelberg grouped themselves benevolently – and this in March 1993, when the accusations against H. M. were just being discussed particularly intensively at the two institutes. E. M. was a victim who had fallen victim to H. M.'s pattern of crimes associated with the psychotherapeutic setting in an almost paradigmatic way. Apart from the director of the adult institute, there seems to have been no one who would have taken responsibility for the young woman. Here, too, it must be argued that this would by no means have been easy or promising, but even in retrospective observation, an attitude of concern for the then very young and biographically burdened woman seems to have been largely absent. E. M. was, so to speak, "lost" in the marriage with the head of the institute, who was still in office at the time, so that the argument of the "private matter" made the question of the institutional assumption of responsibility for the welfare of the young woman seem more or less obsolete.

The pattern of the unequal distribution of responsibility interests was updated in the dynamic described above when there was increasing evidence that H. M. had behaved in a way that was violating sexual boundaries, especially towards boys, in the context of second sights. The described lack of orientation towards the victims can therefore be described quite convincingly as an abdication of responsibility both for the affected boys and for all those people who were and would become patients in H. M.'s practice in Seckach.

From a psychodynamic perspective, it is to be expected that the defence against responsibility in the sense described here triggered feelings of guilt in many actors at various stages of retrospective observation. This raises the question of the extent to which these feelings of guilt were warded off by arguments of appeasement or their appropriateness was critically reflected upon and discussed. We have already seen that a number of conclusive justificatory contexts are available for the defence against such feelings of guilt: Responsibility for oneself, for the children, for the family, for the career, for the institution AKJP-Heidelberg or the institution IPP-Heidelberg-Mannheim. Uncertainty about how to assess the rumours of the time: Relationships between adults, relationships between spouses. Private affairs. Uncertainty about the appropriateness of medical examination practices.

Despite these rational arguments, the discourse on how to deal with the "Causa H. M." was and is filled with mutual accusations of guilt, with feelings of guilt and defended feelings of guilt. Their legitimacy results from the simple fact that H. M. in his function as head of the AKJP-Heidelberg practiced sexual violence for 18 years and afterwards lived in a marriage with a patient, had two children with her and in turn ran a practice for children, adolescents and adults for 18 years, in which all patients were exposed to dangers that could be convincingly derived from H. M.'s past history. It can be stated that most of the persons who could have borne responsibility in this context had successful professional careers, i.e. they fulfilled their responsibility for themselves. It can also be stated that those who assumed responsibility for the continued existence of the institutes AKJP-Heidelberg and IPP-Heidelberg-Mannheim were successful in their efforts in this regard. Finally, it can be stated that we know extraordinarily little about the victims and their fates. The fact that they have remained largely hidden could also be explained by the fact that they did not feel that sufficient responsibility was taken for their well-being and health in the two institutes. Who is to blame for this cannot sensibly be clarified. However, how to deal with associated feelings of guilt can be the subject of further discussion in the context of the two institutes.

The following two sections deal with inner-psychic dynamics and their manifestations, which cannot be seen independently of the described modes of responsibility defense, corresponding feelings of guilt, and the defense against these feelings of guilt.

7.9.2 Forgetting, Denying, Repressing, Not Knowing, Silence

The picture that presents itself to researchers who attempt to systematically reconstruct the "Causa H. M." is initially chaotic. We find contradictions, confusions, omissions, paradoxes, deviations, aberrations and labyrinths. It is the task of the researcher to assemble these fragments into a consistent composition that can claim to provide a frame of reference for further discussion as a coherent narrative. In the third chapter, we have shown by way of example how certain psychological manoeuvres that seemed to be constitutive for dealing with the Causa H. M. are reenacted in the situation of the research interview. These psychological maneuvers deserve a closer look because they have a high explanatory value when one tries to trace the conditions for the emergence, maintenance and lack of working through the past of sexual violence at the AKJP Institute Heidelberg.

We have chosen not to describe various psychological mechanisms separately from one another, but to present them in their interconnectedness. These mechanisms produce – pathetically formulated – symptoms of human imperfection. This is responsible for the fact that we have to rely on piecing together many distorted and incomplete pictures when trying to sketch a consistent picture of the processes at the AKJP-Institut Heidelberg. We acknowledge the error-proneness of reconstructive research, but because we are at the same time in the field of psychoanalysis, we find ourselves reflecting on what contributed to the error-proneness of the information provided to us. In doing so, we recognize that something is reflected in the present that already had decisive effects in those times in which our object of investigation was configured.

On the level of the symptom we first encounter rumours and non-knowledge in many different forms, as can be seen in the following quotation from a psychotherapist:

> *Those are really rumors. So there are a lot of rumors going around, of course. There's a lot of rumors going around and also always this, when he got kicked out and who was involved and who wasn't involved, there's a lot of rumors going around.*

Rumours and not knowing are constitutive concomitants of sexual violence (cf. e.g. Keupp et al. 2017a, 2019). Rumours and non-knowledge create a certain relationship to information. They reconcile an objective proportion of the lack of information with a certain degree of psychological functionality associated with this lack of information. German history has created a paradigm for this psychological functionality of not-knowing, which can be automatically referred to when explaining why it is exculpatory to have (allegedly) had no knowledge of certain facts (Mitscherlich and Mitscherlich 2007).

> *"I didn't know that H. M. had also done something with children" is a figure of argumentation that has achieved some prominence in our study and which has an important function in the sense of the defence against responsibility discussed above. When asked whether, from a retrospective point of view, she/he would behave differently than she/he did at the time, one interviewee answered: "Nope, I don't know. So that I would have the thought that I had missed something, something to do. I didn't have anything to do with children who were affected by him."*

We have also heard this sentence in a similar form from one of the central actors of the inquiry group "Past – Present – Future" (2000). This group was demonstrably initiated, among other things, because reports had accumulated at the Institute that H. M. had committed sexual boundary violations against boys in second sight and examination situations. From this group came – due to indications in the course of the group – the order to search in archives for corresponding records. What does it mean that a protagonist of this group states in the research interview in 2020 that he is now hearing for the first time that H. M. has also committed offences against children? In another interview, a colleague who knew H. M. very well explains that H. M.'s development had taken a perverse, addictive turn, which led him to eventually commit offences against children as well. As long as this was not the case (i.e., as long as this did not need to be known), there was little reason to doubt H. M.'s human and professional integrity (even though it had long been known that he had sexual relations with female patients and teaching analysands).

The functions of non-knowledge are as heterogeneous as its contents: What is it exactly that is not known or may not be known? That H. M. asked boys in the assessment situation whether they were already masturbating? That he touched boys' penises during the medical examination? That he theorized about the connection between existing enuresis and an erection in the examination setting? Knowing this is not threatening, as long as one does not have to describe such episodes in terms of sexual boundary violations. A candidate who only completed her/his training at AKJP-Heidelberg in the 2010s summarizes the non-discourse in this regard as follows:

> *There's a family secret, now I know it too. And then the question is: What do we know? And we didn't really know very much (…). And then I also had the feeling that it was very … that no one could really say – which is also clear (…). But it is also somehow difficult: What is proven, what is not? How do you express it?*

What specifically does the moral horror refer to when one learns in retrospect that H. M. sexually abused children? Nothing is known about H. M. penetrating his young patients anally or making them touch his penis. We only know about his assaultive examination practices, which only condense into a concept of sexual violence when one relates them to his other acts, recognizes the pattern of the narcissistic exercise of power by sexual means, hears the reports of boys and girls who left the examination room deeply ashamed and irritated, and very seriously raises the question of what psychotherapeutic indication should underlie such examination practices.

So what should not be known in order not to endanger the self-concept as a capable psychotherapist and responsible adult too much? One answer might be: "I knew that he touched boys' penises and asked girls about their sexual experiences. But I did not know that he was sexually assaulting boys and girls." The paradoxical nature of this reasoning is immediately obvious, but it likely played and continues to play a major role in the organization of knowledge and the reception of rumors. Evidence of this is the following retrospective formulation from one of our interviews:

> *So occasionally moms would come with kids, or they would come with teenagers, and they would kind of talk about things.*

If one asks what was known in 1992/1993, when the accusations against H. M. were made, a picture of almost complete indifference emerges: "He had relations with former training analysands", "He had a child with a former patient", "He had a child with a patient for the second time", "He had relations with training candidates", "He had committed abstinence violations". It is one of the most striking findings that these fragmentary truths, half-truths or fragments of truths, condensed into rumours, show persistence for decades. It is also interesting that many interview partners are now very uncertain about what H. M. was actually accused of at the time. A labyrinthine circulation of narratives unfolded, which satisfied the recipients' demand to form a judgment. One can assume a psychological defense behind this, whose motive can be described with the formulation "I didn't want to know so exactly". H. M. entered this not entirely unintentional knowledge vacuum offensively by spreading his "subjective truths" about what he was theoretically prepared to place "in the vicinity of abstinence violations". On the fringes of this not entirely unintentional knowledge vacuum were those affected by it, unwilling to fill it with information. Perhaps not enough had been done to increase their readiness in this regard.

The claim that something has to be dealt with here, which for a long time had an emotional impact within the institutes AKJP-Heidelberg and IPP-Heidelberg-Mannheim, still existed decades after H. M.'s resignation from his functions at the institutes. From younger training candidates, who did not know H. M. at all, we learn that the "Causa H. M." is making waves in various segments of the institute environment, whereby the factual basis for these dynamics remains regularly unspecified:

> *That was, I don't know (…), whereby, I don't know at all what he [a former superior from another institution, author's note] told exactly. He said something along the lines of: Well, he must have started something with female patients, and that somehow there was a child and that there were deaths and that he was then thrown out. And so on. But somehow I knew.: There's something there. I didn't know this person, I never saw him.*

This observation is important insofar as it shows that even after many decades, there seems to be no reliable narrative that allows for a purposeful processing of what happened. This is reminiscent of the experiences of members of a Californian psychotherapy institute described by Burka et al. (2019) in the wake of serious ethical breaches at the institute coming to light: "I had no recourse, nowhere to go to make sense of it. Just bits and pieces, fragments here and there, floating in orbit" (p. 258).

In this context, two essential aspects should be pointed out: First, it is in the nature of sexual violence that it takes place mostly in secret and under the seal of secrecy. This is directly evident in the present case, when H. M. exclusively used the exclusive psychotherapeutic or medical setting to initiate and perpetrate his sexual transgressions. A major problem in dealing with sexual violence is often the discrepancy between incomplete information on the one hand and the need for consistent action on the other (Kavemann et al. 2015b). Since many victims remain silent for a variety of serious reasons, this discrepancy, which has many implications, is exacerbated.

The second aspect is particularly interesting because it points directly to sublime psychological functions of not knowing. Since the second half of the 1990s, the later ethics officer of the AKJP-Institute Heidelberg had endeavoured to collect and document available information about the assaults committed by H. M. On the one hand, this caused resistance within the institute, but on the other hand, it was supported by others, for example by the director of the institute, who had been appointed in the meantime. Despite these persistent efforts, which were repeatedly interrupted in the meantime, it was not possible to establish a narrative that would have been recognized as sufficiently well-founded by all actors at the Institute and in its environment. Only the "ZEIT" article fulfilled, at least partially, the function of such a narrative, although, as we could see in our interviews, it was not immune to incomplete reception. Rather, this condensed account of H. M.'s system again triggered in some the reflex of having to protect the Institute from such accusations. One gets the impression that, to this day, no account of H. M.'s deeds has been allowed to develop that could stand a chance of being widely agreed upon, both inside and outside the Institute's public. Burka et al. (2019) report the positive effects of producing a grounded narrative and describe the reaction of Institute members to their report:

> *Those who attended expressed gratitude that so much thinking and metabolizing had transformed disorganized experiences into organized data and conceptual understanding. (p. 260)*

Two opposing movements can be distinguished here: First, the maintenance of the uncertain (and the associated doubting of the empirically grounded) serves to protect an ethically defensible self for some actors. And second, the very incompleteness of information provides an inexhaustible source of psychological stress, conflict, and division. If one does not know with some certainty what the case is, then one tends to fill the gaps in knowledge guided by interests. This leads to the construction of group truths: "Group 'truths' or fantasies emerge to fill in gaps of uncertainty and not-knowing." (Burka et al. 2019, p. 248).

We recognize that (claimed) non-knowledge or half-knowledge in the context of sexual violence is also associated with serious psychological implications, particularly when it relates to an institutional context to which one has belonged or belongs. This is not simply a matter of the availability of information.[9]

In view of these remarks, it becomes understandable why the ethics officers of AKJP-Heidelberg did not succeed in establishing a narrative that would have settled latent and at times burgeoning conflicts at the Institute. Certain versions of the story had to continue to be maintained by certain individuals. This involved both the conscious maintenance of gaps in knowledge ("The people concerned did not report it", "Nothing could be done in terms of criminal law", "It is unclear overall what happened") and the unconscious defence of knowledge with the aim of avoiding feelings of guilt.

This persistence in the unknown has also been passed on to all subsequent years of training. Until today, until the current candidates for training, no narrative has been able to establish itself that speaks of the H. M. era in the institute and its consequences. Some complain about the vagueness, the secrecy, the rumors that spread whisperingly, others share the view, without really being able to name what happened, that disclosure and inquiry only serve to raise the profile of those doing the inquiry and harm the institute. Only in a few interviews did we encounter something like indignation about the sexual boundary violations and those who had held their protective hand over the perpetrator; even more rarely did we encounter empathy for the victims. Thus the patterns of denial, concealment and suppression continue to this day.

A specific form of the production of non-knowledge is forgetting. It is known from many studies, including those relating to sexual violence, that the organization of memory follows a psychological functionality (e.g. Kavemann et al. 2015a; Rieske et al. 2018; Welzer 2002; Welzer et al. 2015). Forgetting by those affected is not only justifiable in terms of trauma theory – in the sense of peritraumatically evoked amnesia – but is also due to pragmatic intentionality (cf. McNally 2005): one forgets facts, for example, because one does not want to think about them, because they have already passed too long, because they were considered too unimportant at the time they happened, or because they happened on a daily basis.

[9] "It's difficult to accept that there is no complete truth or accurate description of a traumatic event (…). When there is no tangible evidence/knowledge of something, akin to a body for grieving, the mind cannot fully comprehend or deal with it (…). Subjected to not-knowing, members are left to develop their own versions of 'truth' that inevitably contain limited information, rumours, and fantasies (…). Individual narratives are affected by unconscious motivations, by the roles members play during investigations, and by their place in the organizational hierarchy. These hybrid narratives can evolve into fixed truths that contribute to conflict in a group" (Burka et al. 2019, p. 265).

The sources of forgetting are numerous and the motivations associated with it diverse.

Describable are numerous variants of forgetting from our interviews: Forgetting the agreed interview date; forgetting times and periods, forgetting important meetings and forgetting names against the background of an interview situation in which one cannot completely distance oneself from the fear that one could denounce fellow human beings, as the following quote from a psychotherapist shows:

> *A: Yes. I noticed during the whole conversation with you that it is simply difficult, so to speak, to give that to the outside.*
> *I: Why do you think it's hard?*
> *A: Yes, because that always has something to do with the fact that you reveal something to someone from your collegial environment. What's right and what you should do, that's what I think. But -*
> *I: I see, but then it's hard.*
> *A: Yes, that is similar to the fact that you don't like to tell from your own family that there are things wrong.*

Forgetting is both the guardian of mistrust and the keeper of information that is better not to be known: Either because one sees one's own self-image endangered or because one anticipates accusations from the interviewer(s) who pledges confidentiality or from a public perceived as threatening. One's experience with the "ZEIT" journalists had not been entirely good.

Since we are in the research field of psychoanalysis, the hermeneutic movement from forgetting to repression is not far away. It is impossible to reconstruct the extent to which information is no longer available primarily because it has fallen victim to an unconscious act of repression that protects one's own self-worth. However, starting points for this assumption can be found: The frequently encountered mode of circulating knowledge delegation, which manifested itself in the fact that interview partners* drew our attention to other persons who ought to know much more. When we interviewed these people, we found that the extent of their knowledge had been overestimated by their colleagues and that they in turn referred to colleagues who supposedly had more knowledge. And so on. A variant of knowledge delegation also consisted in "backpedaling" at the moment when the possibility was opened up that one could take care of the acquisition of further, possibly highly relevant interview partners for the study:

> *A: Even my colleague, who was in supervision with him [H. M., author's note], told me a story that she had with him. But then she broke off the supervision.*

I: (…) Of course we are looking for people who have experienced something like that. So if you could talk to your colleague, if she would be willing to talk to us, that would be great. (…)
A: Yes, but nothing happened, but she told me about an encounter with him where you can understand how that happened.

Another finding is that some interview partners withheld highly relevant information from us, which we were able to unambiguously obtain from other data sources. This in turn goes hand in hand with the observation that such questions were sometimes answered with a "I don't know anymore", the answer to which could possibly have shed a problematic light on one's own involvement in the "Causa H. M.". A further indication for efforts of repression is the recognizable emotional reactions of a part of our interview partners. Some of these persons were surprised themselves that the confrontation with the incidents of that time was associated with such an unexpected emotional involvement even after such a long time.

These statements refer to those persons who were willing to talk to us despite the undeniable threats to their own self-image that were associated with the condensed discussion of the "Causa H. M." in the interview. We also received refusals – from people who "actually did not know H. M. at all", who "could not contribute anything to the matter" or who felt put off by formulations in our data protection statement. And there is a large majority of people involved who did not contact us. That which was not brought to our attention through these variants of silence remains in that realm of institutional repression which is naturally part of any working through the past.

An interesting indication of psychologically motivated ignorance are the years 1991 and 1992, in which H. M. was already living with his young patient, who had given birth to his child in July 1991. This period appears in the reconstruction like a "white spot" in the abundance of information which we were otherwise able to generate on the "Causa H. M.". This information gap is therefore in extreme need of explanation, since in 1991 the child had been born as a visible sign of the sexual relationship between H. M. and his patient. H. M. only felt compelled to launch the lie, according to which the mother was not a patient at all, but a young woman who had merely been presented to him for diagnostic assessment, when critical inquiries were made on the part of the adult institute IPP-Heidelberg-Mannheim on the basis of information from the Youth Welfare Office. The fact that M. P. publicly congratulated the director of the institute, H. M., on the occasion of his 60th birthday and in the context of the 40th anniversary celebration of the institute in the summer of 1992 on his paternity proves that a possibly intended secrecy about the sexual relationship and the child was not successful. In the course of this celebration it was openly discussed that the mother of this child was a patient of H. M. We received this information from an interlocutor who was the only one who spoke about the period between 1991 and 1992. Otherwise: forgetting, repression, not knowing. The child existed, the lavish anniversary celebration with the public congratulation on fatherhood existed, the knowledge circulating in the scene existed that H. M. had a child with a patient. And in the same scene there also existed the knowledge that H. M. had already become the father of a child in 1980, whose mother was another young patient of H. M.'s.

This period from summer 1991 to summer 1992 seems to have been almost completely suppressed from the collective consciousness of the Heidelberg psychotherapy scene. The collective knowledge that existed at that time was retrospectively transformed into a knowledge gap, which was only allowed to take on a changed shape a few months later through the openly and publicly raised accusations of the board of the adult institute IPP-Heidelberg-Mannheim. Now it was denounced that H. M. had sexually exploited female teaching analysts as well as impregnated a female patient. While the newly-born father had been applauded at the summer party, the same facts suddenly became part of a worrying scandal that threatened the existence of the institute, the training of many candidates, the jobs of some staff members and the reputation of many psychotherapists. Around the birth of the child in 1991, a more or less involved public of therapists had gathered, who, as far as we know, could not find anything objectionable about H. M.'s relationship with the young patient. Thus, from a psychodynamic point of view, it is not surprising that this period remains completely underrepresented, unmentioned, i.e. repressed in all narratives. The discourse does not begin until the end of 1992/beginning of 1993, and a certain faction in the institute and in its environment does not allow itself to be prevented from attending the wedding celebration of the two in March 1993, from acting as maid of honor, and a little later from welcoming the birth of the second child by the scandalization of facts that have become known in the meantime. None of this can be put into language later, and it is left to reflexive speculation whether this results from forgetting, repression, denial, or the deliberate misappropriation of information.

This "white spot" on the map of the narratives about the "Causa H. M." is by no means unusual. It refers to a whole series of situations and facts which were described to us in a confusing and contradictory manner. Indeed, based on these observations, the image of an "institutional dissociation" can be endeavored, as described by Burka et al. (2019) in their analysis of a similar case in the United States. As a symptom of such a dissociative representation of the institutional past, they identify a perceptual habitus they call "fogginess". This term immediately resonates with us when we become aware of the difficulties in attempting to gather consistent data and information about the past of the Heidelberg AKJP Institute. Confusions about dates, names, and facts appear as a symptom of something unprocessed, as an expression of dissociative fogginess, and not simply as a problem of an "objective" lapse of memory in the face of long-ago periods.

Silence is a constitutive concomitant of sexual violence. It fulfils important psychological and social functions for the victims as well as for the perpetrators and possible confidants. That silence helps the perpetrators is a very abbreviated statement, even if it is not entirely factually incorrect, but at best it is suitable as a campaign slogan and thus as a morally charged appeal. In the present case, in various phases of the conflictual dispute about H. M., things came to a head which ultimately reduced the problem to this mechanism: the fact that neither the teaching analysands affected nor the young patient E.M. were prepared to speak to law enforcement agencies or health insurance companies about the exact circumstances of the initiation of the respective sexual relationships with H. M. meant that it was not possible to take action against H. M. with the necessary consistency. The functions of this silence do not need further explanation: The fear of losing the good reputation as a psychotherapist in Heidelberg; the shame about the fact that one's own intimate life could become the subject of disputes in the context of a public that could not be controlled and – on the part of E. M. – the fear of losing all existential foundations that were tied to the marriage with H. M.

An important psychological function of silence is that the naming of facts is always linked to the creation of reality (Keupp et al. 2019). By finding its way into the "language game" (in Wittgenstein's sense), something becomes part of a world that is everything "that is the case" (Wittgenstein and Kenny 1996). This aspect is far from trivial, because it contributed over years and decades to the fact that H. M.'s sexual transgressions did not "exist" as such in the context of asymmetrical power relations. In fact, the accusations from the adult institute IPP-Heidelberg-Mannheim changed the language game at the end of 1992. This significantly limited the possibilities of undoing through silence. But it cannot be said that silence did not continue to retain its subjectively useful function for many of those involved.[10]

Silence means: not subjecting the subjective representations of one's own body of knowledge to social validation. Silence is the social practice that provides a secure framework for the unreliable inner-psychic maneuvers of repression, denial, and reinterpretation. Each interview in the context of our research project therefore also represented a form of self-exposure. This was associated with certain psychological risks, especially for contemporary witnesses who still knew H. M. personally: "And I know that for many – I spoke with a colleague who was also very involved at the time. I wrote to her and also forwarded her the information that you wanted to conduct these interviews. And she said she couldn't do it. So there are also many where that is so lastingly traumatic to this day."

Discursive deconstruction of one's own version of an emotionally occupied past. To speak means: to put one's own constructions at disposal, to take emotional risks. All psychotherapists know this. They know the superficially useful functions of silence, which, however, have the inherent problem of inhibiting development. And they know the risks and the potentials of speaking.

There are many variants of silence, some of which we got to know in the course of our study, for example the sudden change of topic in an interview with a psychotherapist:

> *I: Did you hear any rumours about H. M. at the Institute, were there – because there were some who said, yes, it was known here that he had relationships with female teaching analysts?*
>
> *A: Yes, that already seeped through, but now from the theoretical situation, I find it so interesting, his attitude to psychoanalysis.*

Obvious omissions or the ability to speak so softly that blanks appear in the interview transcript in just such answers that referred to particularly important questions represent further possibilities of concealment. There is a wide range of what cannot be collected in the context of such a study. There is much that remains untold. And there is a sense that it is in what has not been told that there may be par-

[10] On the functions and consequences of silence in a similar context, Burka et al. (2019) write: "Silencing is ubiquitous in institutes after the revelation of a boundary violation. We might ask: is silencing in the service of survival, an attempt to prevent further chaos in response to an analytic treatment gone out of control? Or is silencing in the service of negation, an attempt to cope by relying on a cover-up? When silencing is used defensively, it stimulates further disruption, as members feel overly managed or excluded. In silence, members are left to manage an incomprehensible event without benefit of discourse or community care" (p. 264).

ticularly much and fundamental information. This is also something that is very familiar to all psychoanalytically thinking and working people: the actual that is hidden in what is not said. On the level of behavioural manifestation one could also say: Some who would have had something to say did not talk to us, as we explicitly learn from the interview with a psychotherapist:

> *I don't know exactly how, but the [colleague, author's note] said to me the other day – I have a coffee with her now and then – she said, yes, I could really tell you a lot. But that is also subject to the rule of secrecy. I believe that she had someone – one or two people in analysis or therapy who were actually affected. She herself is certainly not affected by it].*

Hypotheses can be made about the silence of those who have not spoken to us. What is most striking here is the silence of the victims. Working through the past of sexual violence in an institutional context requires the voices of the victims (Mosser et al. 2018; Unabhängige Aufarbeitungskommission 2019b). In the present case, these voices have to be largely dispensed with, although it is imperative to view this state of affairs as symptomatic. In addition to all the well-known reasons that prevent people who have been affected by sexual violence from speaking about their experiences, two aspects that are likely to be particularly characteristic of sexual violence in the context of psychotherapy should be mentioned at this point:

First, the exclusive, individualized setting of psychotherapeutic treatment makes it difficult to organize the victims after the fact. This is immediately understandable when one contrasts sexual violence in, for example, convent boarding schools or schools. Although there are pronounced structures of secrecy in such institutional settings as well, there is nevertheless something like a common everyday atmosphere to which those affected can also refer in retrospective observation. They know each other and, to a certain extent, they also know about each other, so that there are possibilities to form as a group in order to jointly denounce violence suffered (Mosser and Straus 2020). Such possibilities are not available to the psychotherapy patient treated in the context of individual therapy. There is usually no contact between outpatients, especially since the use of psychotherapy was associated with strong feelings of shame, as one of the psychotherapists we interviewed confirmed:

> *After all, it wasn't often said in the old days that people went to therapy. It was one of the best-kept secrets, along with bed-wetting.*

Secondly, H. M.'s sexual boundary violations did not only refer to children and adolescents, but also to adults. We are dealing here with constellations of offenses that are very difficult to assign conceptually, even in retrospect. If we consider the definition of sexual violence by Bange and Deegener (1996) mentioned earlier, the problem becomes immediately understandable because it is based on the fact that the sexual act is carried out against the will of a child or that "the child cannot knowingly consent due to physical, psychological, cognitive or linguistic inferiority." Most adult victims in H. M.'s case will not be able to assert these criteria. In most cases, there will also have been no direct use of violence, so that the victims were and are faced with the extraordinarily challenging task of generating a coherent inner concept of their experiences that is not completely overburdened by feelings of shame and guilt. In the course of our studies, we spoke with many people who had often experienced (sexual) violence in an institutional context many decades earlier. Although they were children or adolescents at the time, some of them still find it difficult to cope with feelings of shame and complicity today (Caspari et al. 2021; Keupp et al. 2017a, b, 2019). For most, however, it is clear that they were sexually exploited as minors at the time – as defined by Bange and Deegener (1996). For the adult victims in the case of H. M., on the other hand, it is much more difficult to distance themselves from the assessment that the sexual acts were "voluntary" and "consensual" and that one could just as well have said "no". One interviewee expressed this as follows:

> *It's not rape, he doesn't lay her on the couch against her will. But this is – there is an erotic relationship network, in which the patient or the patient enters voluntarily, in inverted commas.*

Only a comprehensive understanding of the entire case with its highly complex power-dependency dynamics should be able to contribute to reliably saying goodbye to such self-harming cognitions.

We do not know how many of the victims have spoken about their experiences with H. M. in the context of psychotherapies, counselling or in their private environment. We can only state that within the framework of the research project – with one exception – no women came forward who had been involved in sexual interactions or relationships with H. M. as adults. At least, our female interviewees did not speak of this. However, the fact that some women reported that H. M. "was not interested in me", that "I did not fit into his pattern" or that "he should not have tried it with me" has explanatory value because it refers to what is easier to say. This is what a psychotherapist said in an interview:

Well, I am someone who is very clearly defined, very clearly structured, and that's how I appear. H. M. would never have dared in a hundred years, in his simple primitiveness on a certain level – he would never have dared to cross a boundary, because he felt that it was simply not possible.

Implicit in this is why other women have not spoken to us.

Against this background, the few reports of the victims who suffered sexual-boundary violations by H. M. as a child or adolescent are of particular value for the analysis presented here. They give us unequivocal information about the way in which H. M. exploited psychotherapeutic or assessment situations in order to sexually exploit people. They also contain convincing information about the emotional reactions these assaults provoked in the victims and how strongly they continued to have an effect, in part, later on.

The large area of the unsaid includes the silence of those affected and it includes the silence of contemporary witnesses, i.e. former training candidates, employees and managers at the institutes IPP-Heidelberg-Mannheim and AKJP-H eidelberg. The motives and the contents of this silence naturally remain in the realm of the speculative, even if we receive some meaningful hints, e.g. from an interviewed psychotherapist:

A: Well, that is also the defense of the repressed, I say. I feel the same way, when I talk about it now, I think, uh, now I've told you about Mrs. X, she was also with me in the intervision group, she lives in my street, yes, I'll denounce her now. Mechanisms like that come up, they are specific for such things, yes, that you then think, are you betraying someone now? So. (…) No, it's not that simple.

So from a data protection point of view, of course, you are protected, and yet I notice how I withhold information, I'll put it that way. (laughs) (…) No, I have – I mean, what I say here is really data-protected. We met Ms. Y after the trial. My colleagues and I. But that is now – I also have data protection [mumbles unintelligibly] so I mean, I don't know now how much I can say.

I: You have to decide.

A: Yes. (Pause) Yes, we got a lot of information from that side anyway.

With regard to the function of silence, it is important to remember the basic dynamic between functional pragmatism on the one hand and the thematization of sexual violence at AKJP-Heidelberg on the other. In some interviews it becomes apparent that exposing oneself to questioning researchers is also exposing oneself to partially burdening memories and that in this way the mode of functional pragmatism is at least partially abandoned: "Now I realize how crazy the whole thing is or how much I have repressed it!"

In the meantime we can say that in different phases of the history of the Institute it was "reasonable" to remain silent. There are many people who were entangled by H. M. in a system of dependence, but also of unconscious or careless complicity. This necessitates the defense of embarrassing loyalties and omissions that become apparent after the fact. The renunciation of a social negotiation of such entanglements can contribute to the maintenance of a (unconsciously) threatened psychological stability and action-related functionality.

Forgetting, repression, denial, not knowing and silence form a complex of defence mechanisms and symptoms which are characteristic for the handling of the "Causa H. M." at the AKJP-Institute Heidelberg. The list of manifestations we observed, which can be described within the framework of psychoanalytic terminology, could be continued: Blame attributions, defense against feelings of guilt, aggressive defense, rationalization, dissociative confusion, … From a psychodynamic point of view, it can be stated that the "Causa H. M." has apparently been processed up to the present day to an extent that can be associated with the emergence of such manifestations. The fact that in all phases of the development of the institute the defense against such a processing was experienced by more or less large factions within the AKJP-Heidelberg as reasonable and sensible, is above all in need of explanation, because the analogies to a psychoanalytical understanding of human processes impose themselves unmistakably. If one sees conflicts and emotional charges as indications of processing requirements, then it seems to be necessary in various phases of the development of even a psychoanalytic institution to leave the path of functional pragmatism and to expose oneself.

7.10 Groups and Conflicts

In the following, an attempt will be made to provide an overview of the complex events of conflict that have been grouped around the "Causa H. M." since the disclosures at the end of 1992/1993 at the latest. This is done here in a deliberately simplified manner in order to enable a basic understanding of the roles of the instances involved. Simplifications are always associated with considerable loss of information. Nevertheless, at this point we initially choose the form of graphical representation that can be related to the dynamics described in the previous and subsequent chapters (Fig. 7.2). The graph is intended to illustrate a rough location of the instances involved across four different developmental phases of the AKJP Institute Heidelberg. When interpreting the diagram, it is important to bear in mind that the groups involved were not themselves amorphous or completely homogeneous, but that they were mostly represented by certain protagonists who were

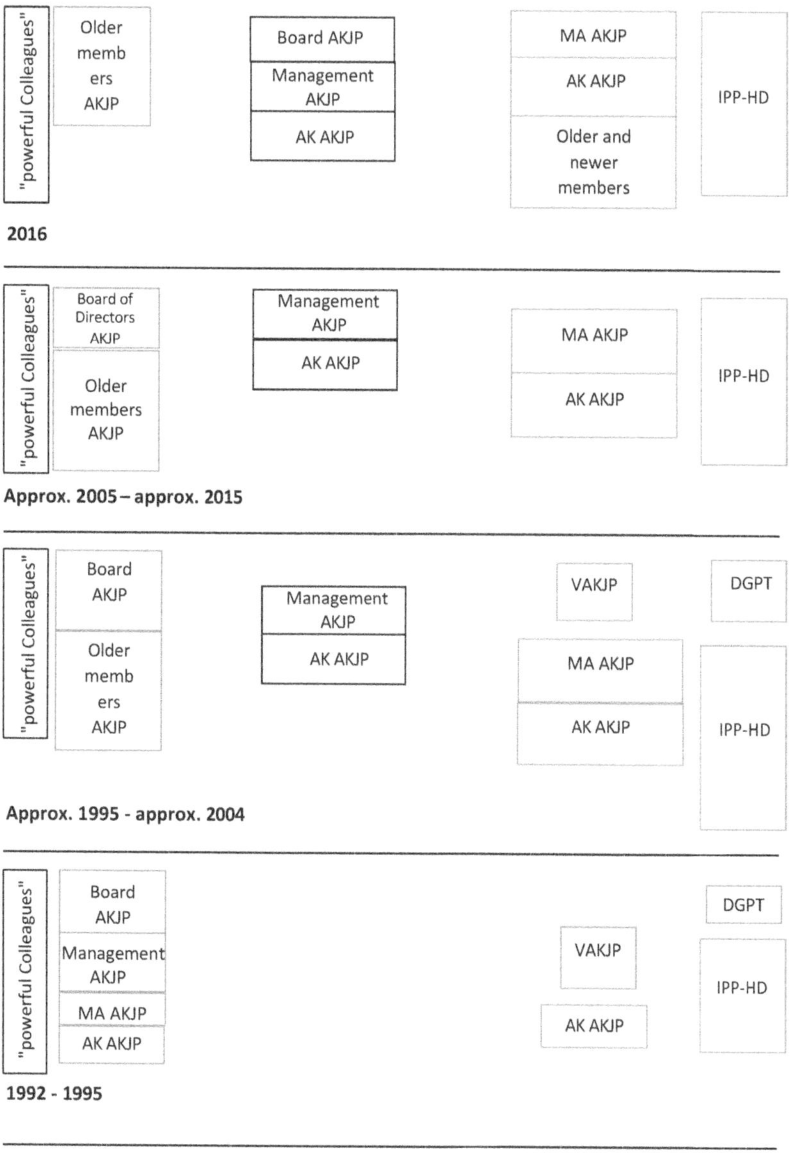

Fig. 7.2 Conflict fractions. Abbreviations: *AK* Ausbildungskanditat*innen (training candidates), *MA* Mitarbeiter*innen (staff members). (Own representation)

more or less strongly associated with a greater or lesser number of allies. The left area of the graph symbolizes those instances that followed the mode of functional pragmatism described above and/or actively sought to cover up the accusations against H. M.. The right area indicates those instances that sought to clarify the incidents, to speak about the problem and to work through the past for the long term. In between are those who could not take a clear position – either because they could not or did not want to know anything about the "Causa H. M." or because they were entangled in discrepant loyalties.

The following facts can be derived from the graph:

In the context of the accusations in 1993, it can be said that the AKJP-Institute Heidelberg took a stance of defending its institute director on almost all levels. Exceptions to this are those approx. 5 training candidates who – with the support of the VAKJP – demanded clarification and H. M.'s resignation.

In the further course, especially on the board level and at least partially on the staff level, forces were still represented that were loyal to H. M. and undermined efforts to clarify and inquire the situation. These were more or less strongly associated with "powerful colleagues" in the Heidelberg psychotherapy scene.

The adult institute IPP-Heidelberg-Mannheim remained an authority throughout the entire period, from which impulses for inquiry emanated at irregular intervals.

Within the AKJP-Heidelberg, attempts at clarification and inquiry were initiated primarily by individual employees with occasional support from training candidates.

The management of the AKJP-Heidelberg, which was appointed in 1994, remained neutral. From the management level, efforts to clarify the situation were supported in principle, but without identifying and isolating those forces which continued to be loyal to H. M. and remained quite influential at the institute.

It is striking that the basic structure with regard to the positioning of the conflicting parties has remained largely unchanged over decades. This is also related to the fact that the main protagonists of the (more or less latently conducted) disputes also remained unchanged over long periods of time. This does not rule out the possibility that there were movements within the individual factions that went hand in hand with changes in their respective spheres of influence.

In accordance with what we have said so far and what will be presented below, we can speak of an enduring conflict that is explicitly represented by individual persons, but which at the same time has shaped the entire development of the Institute in phases up to the present day. These phases can be described as a succession of violently updatedevents of conflict on the one hand and "asymptomatic latency periods" on the other (see also Chap. 8). It can be said that since 1993 there has been no one in the AKJP-Heidelberg and in the environment of the Institute who has not been caught up in these more or less subterranean currents of conflict. The conflict did not cease to exist, even if one can speak of a relatively calm latency phase, especially for the period from about 2005 to about 2016, which was, however, abruptly ended by the criminal charges against H. M., the subsequent court proceedings and the publication of the "ZEIT" article.

We have described several dynamics and motivations that gave rise to the persistent lines of conflict at the AKJP Institute in Heidelberg:

Endangering the existence of the institute, endangering the existential foundations of many staff members and training candidates, personal entanglements and loyalties with H. M., enduring power and dependency relationships, resistance to the topic of "sexual violence" and fear of confrontation with victimization and victims, resistance to responsibility towards the victims in favour of a perception of responsibility for oneself and the institute, denial, repression, forgetting, silence.

It has been worked out that the modes of reaction described have a tendency to affect each other reciprocally, whereby violent counter-reactions can be triggered both at the level of the subject and at the level of the institution: The latent mode of cover-up, masked by the attitude of functional pragmatism, finds itself immediately threatened the moment "the old subject" is brought back to the surface of the institution-related discourse by any side. Conversely, the propagation of downplaying or ignoring narratives triggers reactances in those persons who are convinced that the "Causa H. M." has still not been sufficiently dealt with. Symptomatically, this dynamic is primarily associated with the attribution of guilt, with the emergence of feelings of guilt and the defence against them.

In the context of our study, one interviewee reported on a conversation following the general meeting of the AKJP-Heidelberg, which dealt with the decision to commission a scientific study to investigate the "Causa H. M.". She/he had experienced the general meeting itself as very emotionally charged. In the subsequent dialogue with a representative of the AKJP Institute Heidelberg, they also talked about the role of H. M.'s daughter, who had made a very significant contribution to the clarification of his sexual boundary violations– also at the AKJP Heidelberg – with the criminal complaint against her father. Her/his interlocutor had expressed appreciation for the role of this daughter, which led our interviewee to the following reaction:

"And even I, who I am after all thoughtful, said, now stop heroizing the victims!" So I thought, what am I saying? Can I hear myself say that? I thought, "What a stupid thing to say. You get so aggressive! Or you get defensive. And what goes around comes around, you wake up at night."

In this short sequence, much is described in a condensed form, which we were also able to work out from many other interviews. Some motives become recognizable, to which a high explanatory value for the persistent character of the conflict dynamics prevailing at AKJP-Heidelberg can be attributed. First of all, we have to take into account the fact that the conversation reported by the interviewee took place in 2019, i.e. 25 years after the partial disclosure of H. M.'s sexual boundary violations, which led to his resignation as head of the institute.

The emotional vehemence associated with the discursive reactualization of the event is unmistakable. Even the character trait of "thoughtfulness", which is otherwise experienced as reliable, is suspended in the face of the interviewee's words of appreciation for H. M.'s daughter. It is unbearable for the interviewee that in this way "the victims are heroicized". It seems reasonable to assume that the perceived "heroization" of the victim (which in the formulation used is equated with a heroization of all victims) endangers the defence against one's own feelings of guilt: Theultimately successful criminal complaint filed by H.M.'s daughter drew effects that made the extent of the failures of all actors at the psychotherapy institutes obvious. The child, born in 1993, finally had to take the step that the Heidelberg psychotherapist community had been unable to take for 25 years: well-founded criminal charges, credible testimony, criminal and thus publicly perceptible disclosure of the sexual acts of violence with subsequent conviction. This act of H. M.'s daughter holds up a mirror especially to those persons from his environment who knew him well and worked with him: Ignoring circumstantial evidence, trivializing his boundary transgressions, retreating to alleged or actual ignorance. We don't know what our interviewee sees in that mirror, but something in her/him reminds her/him of failings that taint her/him with guilt. We cannot assess to what extent these feelings of guilt are due to real and obvious failures. What is important, however, is the symptomatic vehemence of the emotional response triggered by the words of appreciation for H. M.'s daughter. Whether someone who reports her own father for sexual abuse needs to be "heroized" is not the question – such behavior is certainly worthy of recognition. Our interviewee, however, is outraged by this recognition. She/he asks her/his interlocutor to stop. She/he obviously can't hear it anymore, because something inside her/him gets into an almost unbearable turmoil.

The special thing about the further description is the self-reflexive moment. The interviewee comes out of his/her shell and expresses astonishment about the reaction just shown. It can be assumed that this self-reflective moment has usually remained underrepresented in the real conflicts between the factions represented in AKJP-Heidelberg. The averted feeling of guilt usually led to aggressive acting out ("You get so aggressive!"), which naturally leads to corresponding reactions on the other side: Deflected feeling of guilt, aggressive response, attribution of guilt, defense against feelings of guilt, etc. – the paradigm of conflict dynamics at the AKJP Institute Heidelberg. This is further illustrated by the sentence: "Or one becomes defensive". In fact, the interviewee was not reproached in any way by her/his interlocutor. The person only referred to the merits of H. M.'s daughter. This does not represent an intended attack on her/his former behaviour, but obviously triggers massive reactions on an unconscious level, which immediately cause one to "become defensive".

The self-reflexive moment consists of wondering about oneself. It is not clear from this interview sequence to what extent the interviewee has an explanation for his/her reactions. First of all, however, the perception of one's own astonishment alone is remarkable. The question arises as to what causes one to refuse to acknowledge a courageous young woman who has reported her sexually abusive father. It remains unclear what the interviewee wakes up to at night. Something is seriously undone. Something reminds us again and again of inner conflicts and urges us to act on them externally. We also feel reminded of all that was said above about the consistent turning away from the victims. Any confrontation with the fact that there were victims seems to threaten one's psychological and ethical integrity. That there were victims reminds us that there were acts that victimized others. But this also reminds us of our own responsibility, which would have been to prevent or name these acts, or at least to enter into a serious, careful and process-oriented discourse with others about relevant circumstantial evidence.

H. M.'s daughter, whose daughter was sexually abused by H. M., functions in this narrative as a cipher for all persons who have fallen victim to H. M. s acts. Mentioning them is equated with their "heroization" in the guilt-ridden perception. One could also say: Whoever talks about the victims heroizes them. In doing so, the heroization is discursively easier to ward off than the simple fact that they are mentioned and that recognition is given to them.

Turning to the fate of the victims involves the risk of being reminded of one's own failings. At this point, no statements can be made about real failures on the part of our interview partner. What is important here is above all what her/his narrative contributes to the explanation of the enduring, violent conflict dynamics at AKJP-Heidelberg. It can be assumed that many protagonists of this conflict did not take the step that is so impressively described by the colleague described here: The conscious questioning of the self, the astonishment at what one has just said, and the pressing nature of those questions that rob one of sleep. It can be assumed that the processing and coping culture of AKJP-Heidelberg has left too little room for such self-reflexive processes.

Therefore, certain information, assessments, opinions, narratives functioned again and again as triggers for impulse-driven reactions, which gave rise to corresponding emotional counter-reactions. Again and again, the admission had to be fought off that people had been harmed by H. M.'s sexual boundary violations, in part severely, and that one had possibly not sufficiently perceived the responsibility for these people and for all those who had been harmed by him at a later time. How "real" these failures were and how "justified" the associated feelings of guilt are can only be found out within the framework of individual and institutional processes of working through the past, which are free of mutual recriminations and existential threat scenarios.

7.11 Exemplary Case Reconstructions

In order to illustrate some of the aspects elaborated in the previous chapters in more detail, two interview partners (Ms/Mr. A. and Ms./Mr. B.) will be compared in the following. Both were employees (lecturers and supervisors respectively) of the AKJP-Institute under H. M. for a long time, and they were also directly on site and involved in the process at the time of the disclosure in 1993. This may be one reason why both show a specific pattern of defensiveness. In contrast to the individuals who declined to participate in the study on the grounds that they did not want to rehash everything after such a long time, felt that they were too affected, or judged such late investigation to be nonsensical, the two individuals wanted their perspective of caveat to be represented in the study. In the following, a third interview partner (Ms/Mr. C.), who was also sceptical about the study but nevertheless was willing to be interviewed, will be included in the evaluation.

The interview partners presented here unanimously show a certain inner tension of conflict between different lines of argumentation: A renewed debate would have no benefit. The financial expenditure for the Institute could not be justified. There is a risk of lasting damage to the Institute's reputation. On the other hand, however, we don't want to be seen as obstructors again, and we want to use the opportunity to refute internal and explicitly expressed accusations that we experience both latently and directly.

The perceived inner reproach of having overlooked something, of not having dealt with it sufficiently, of having missed something and not having done enough, becomes very clear in the two interviews initially considered here. Both persons defend their attitude and their position at the time, but there are discernible differences in the course of the interviews: While the first interviewee insists on her/his defensive position, in the second interview the interviewee's attitude changes in that the latent accusation of insinuation becomes explicit and thus a process of confrontation can be named, even though the main line of expediency of one's own actions is not fundamentally abandoned.

It is conceivable that the strategy of persistent defence in the first case is due to the format of the telephone interview and that this did not reduce the mistrust towards the interviewer. Another reason for the consistent maintenance of one's own position could be the greater involvement of the interviewee in the events of the time.

Among other things, due to the dependence of psychotherapists at that time on the medical delegation procedure, both interview partners can be shown to have constellations that had the character of one of those superficial win-win situations that H. M. often created. At first this is not to be questioned further. However, when it comes to the question of who had something to lose by "unmasking" H. M. or who had something to cover up, such a constellation becomes somewhat explosive. One interviewee reported about quite uncomplicated delegation appointments with H. M., which were associated with little effort for all participants, but took place outside of the structures intended for this purpose. The other interview partner describes that she was able to use the rooms of the institute for her training at the adult institute.

I: And that's where you treated the adults?

A: Yes. And then I sat behind them on my chair, and there I treated the adults, which was a bit embarrassing for me, because it was a bit very unorthodox.

Basically, this exemplary "concession" by the head of the institute is not reprehensible, even if it is certainly more than "a bit very unorthodox". It represents a clear privilege that she/he could use the rooms and possibly also complete parts of her/his training during her/his working hours. At first this seems like a friendly move on the part of the head of the institute, but in this way internal and external dependencies are created.

Through these forms of accommodation on the part of H. M., contours of a system of dependency become visible. H. M. grants privileges – whether willingly or implicitly, whether consciously or unconsciously – in a framework that does not conform to the rules and is almost illegal. Such violations of rules can be classified as not further dramatic in themselves, so that one could "turn a blind eye". This is also against the background that, for example, the medical delegation of psychotherapy for trained psychoanalysts was not uncontroversial and was later also abolished. A violation of the rules in this respect would therefore have been easily reconciled with one's own ideas, according to which this unnecessary procedure should "actually" be circumvented. But with such slight transgressions, a system is quickly created by which one involuntarily enters a legal grey area and ultimately becomes susceptible to blackmail, even if this is not made explicit. This may play a role in the question whether one places oneself critically towards H. M. after accusations against him have become known or stands by him (at first).

One interviewee describes his own attitude towards the rumours at the institute as follows:

So that was my thing, I figured it's none of my business, like he doesn't know who I'm marrying either, so it's none of my business for now. Yes.

Mrs./Mr. A also said:

... and I didn't hear about any of this – so it wasn't until this was cooking – so I didn't hear about any of these machinations.

At the beginning of 1993 a meeting of the members of the adult institute IPP-Heidelberg-Mannheim is prepared, in which H. M. is to be expelled from the institute. Abstinence violations were given as the reason. These are not specified in the meeting. H. M. escapes the confrontation and the expulsion by resigning from his functions at the IPP-Heidelberg-Mannheim beforehand. Both interview partners initially see him as the "attacked" one who is thrown out of the adult institute. While Ms./Mr. B. hardly knows anything official, Ms./Mr. A. comments on this as follows:

I: How did you first hear that there were accusations against H. M.?

A: I can't tell you all that exactly anymore. But I heard, presumably through the head of the institute, that there was now this – yes, now one must first say so. So H. M. – it's difficult to reconstruct, H. M. had in the time when he was still head of the institute – it came out that he had had an affair with a young female patient. And then in Heidelberg, through the Youth Welfare Office, charges were filed, etc. And H. M. got ahead of the whole thing by marrying this young woman.

Not many of those we interviewed knew where the initiative to disclose the boundary violations came from. Most of them had knowledge of the assaults on the teaching analysts at the IPP-Heidelberg-Mannheim, but these were not named for reasons of confidentiality, whereby the explanation that ultimately adults "had something together" here quickly led to a legitimization and weakening of the accusations.

However, it was the Youth Welfare Office that had received news of possible sexual abuse at the institute. The authority already knew about the first illegitimate son of H. M. with a patient and was concerned about the birth of another child of another patient. It is surprising, however, that the institutes IPP-Heidelberg-Mannheim and AKJP-Heidelberg were alarmed only when this patient was already pregnant for the second time by H. M. in 1993. Mrs./Mr. A.:

> *And with the young, with the new Mrs. M., that's true, there was then, after – but then I already had nothing more to do with it. So there was sometime after the first child, there was sometime later again a second girl.*

Thus questions remain open in the interview: Did nobody at the institute know anything about the liaison of the patient with H. M. before 1993, especially since she had the first child in 1991? Also the fact that he had an illegitimate son had not been questioned before. Mrs./Mr. A.:

> *I never wondered from whom. It wouldn't have occurred to me either. I knew he was looking after this son. Z. was his name. Yes. It was important to me that he'd take care of him. "Otherwise I thought he'd be funny with women."*

In the interview with Ms./Mr. A. it is noticeable that the interviewee initially answers only hesitantly, almost as in an interrogation, and in each case only to what is previously stated as known. This pattern, characterized by piecemeal concessions and partial "concessions", is found again and again in an interview that is not an accusation, but which is probably inwardly perceived as such. Thus, the argumentation figure is also brought forth that H. M. had "forestalled" the difficulties that the Youth Welfare Office could have caused him by marrying the patient. This view, through which the case seems to be "settled" for the interviewee and which initially remains completely uncommented, is questioned again by the interviewer.

However, the interviewee continues to accept H. M.'s strategy of appeasement: There is a problem that needs to be solved on a factual level. The interviewee does not further problematize what it actually means when the head of the institute has two children with a young patient. This pragmatism throughout the interview seems to reflect a certain mode of dealing with H. M.'s behaviour at the institute. Both interview partners are primarily concerned with the continued existence of the Institute. This is the line of reasoning on a functional level: It must continue. Behind this it can be assumed that a deeper confrontation could also make visible one's own entanglement (here by not questioning or looking away or by "letting live and let live"). This would be explicable by the latent dependencies described above. Mrs./Mr. B.:

You were just totally shocked at first. Shocked. And that was actually the case, he was gone, and it was unclear what was going to happen to the institute. It was completely open. There were training candidates who were in the middle of their training. Then final exams had to be taken, nobody was there anymore (laughs). That was very, very difficult. Difficult.

The question of how to proceed with the Institute was initially a very concrete and practical question, but at the same time it overshadowed and sometimes obscured the internal movements of the inquiry. This concern not only applies to the phases of disclosure and the subsequent transition, but we also encounter it again and again in the current interviews. The third interviewee presented here (Ms/Mr. C.) explains right at the beginning of the interview why she/he views our study with concern:

The fact that all this costs a lot of money and that a rather small association, that it would ... and the probability that this study is enough, is not so great, I guess, but that there would be new (...) at some point. So my worst fear would be that the institute is ruined, also financially and in terms of the name. And actually I would rather have them do their work, and independently gain clarity or a clarification, processing, because that is certainly a very difficult story and a difficult task.

This pragmatic justification is later supported by reference to the fate of the Odenwald School, but it also testifies to a fundamental resistance to a working through the past:

So that's the death of any institute, like the death of the Odenwald School.

Feeling committed to the continued existence of the institute is a narrative that, according to our information, was also frequently used by A. A. in particular, in order to avoid having to confront the issue further.

It may be a coincidence that the recording quality of Ms./Mr. C's interview is very poor, so that many passages remained difficult to understand. Perhaps the refusal of a clear positioning is expressed here. In any case, the mode of soft speaking and unclear expression contributes to leaving much in the dark. This impression is quite clear from the analysis of the interview with Mrs./Mr. C.

All three interviewees presented here seemed to feel more or less prejudiced by our investigation, reluctant to disclose information, as if every piece of information carried a moral charge and an emotional burden.

Another conspicuous feature in the interviews analysed here was that many names and events were no longer remembered. In principle, this is not surprising after such a long time. What seemed to us to be in need of explanation was rather the way in which forgetting was dealt with succinctly.

Ms./Mr. A., for example, seems reluctant to admit more than is necessary. The conversation often follows the pattern of "quid pro quo", in which the interviewee only confirms what the interviewer has already stated as information.

An interview would offer the opportunity to present certain events once again from a retrospective, whereby it would also be possible to reflect on the motives one had at the time and how one evaluates them from today's perspective. In the interviews presented here, however, the attitude still seems to be one of avoidance, although the interviewees had actively agreed to participate in the study.

However, as described above, forgetting and incomplete memories are not only characteristics of the group studied here, but these phenomena are also found in other interviews. This leads us to the conclusion that there is no narrative in the sense of a narrative within the public of the institute that could have been formed through frequent verbalization and regular exchange. Narratives that are readily reported experience a different emphasis. The accounts presented to us tend to be encountered in a fractured form. The interviewees speak softly and seem forgetful. An exception in this regard are individual persons from the group of training candidates from H. M.'s time, who were directly affected by the upheaval in 1993 and already experienced themselves as speakers at that time, but were not heard. Later training candidates, who were not directly involved in the events, were more willing to provide information and more open than actors from earlier generations.

As already mentioned, through verbalization the experience becomes a narrative and thus a subjective truth. At the same time, this fulfils the claim of a psychotherapeutic attitude that makes processing possible. However, forms of naming and discussing that have been practiced so far do not seem to have created clarity, despite the attempts at processing that have been described. Here is an excerpt from an interview with Mrs./Mr. A.:

I: Did you feel that at some point there was clarity about what H. M. was doing?
A: Yes. So how that – so it was, it was clear that, that, that with the boys – that at some point it was just clear that there had been these sexual assaults with female teaching analysts. But not at our institute.
I: Well, I don't want to declare it right away, but according to all we know, there were sexual relationships with female students at your institute.
A: Good. That's something I don't know. And I hear now also from you for the first time.

It fits in with this that parallels to H. M.'s "theory" of the analogue level in play therapy became apparent in some interviews. The analogue level means that one meets the child exclusively on the level of action and avoids verbalising the experience. Certain institutional narratives also reveal processing patterns that remain on the level of action, as is clear from the following interview quotation (Ms/ Mr. A.):

> *So what I – I was, as I said, for a long time [in the position] – and how then through all this – through processing, that is, psychodynamic processing the restructuring of the institute, the nest-building, that the institute was bought, etc., was my very certain experience, the thing was pacified.*

Other interviews (here: Ms./Mr. C.) also refer to the move to another building and the associated symbolic reinvention of the Institute:

> *There's also this committee that meets once a year and discusses finances or (...) what was still discussed for a while, which was always to sell this little house they had over there and now, where they are now, to take rent there. Now that was a tiny house, a real witch's cottage. With dark rooms and terribly cramped, seminar room, and then the idea was, (...), that's what A. A. already did that. And with that, H. M. was also eliminated to some extent.*

The narrative figure presented here is possibly meant to suggest that a "cleansed" new beginning was made possible by a new house, a new white on the walls. This desire to leave something burdensome behind seems perfectly understandable within the framework of an "analogue" understanding of inquiry. However, such a view is certainly not analytical.

Another narrative figure, which was not only produced in the group under closer examination here, refers to the marginal character of one's own position: one actually did not have that much to do with all this. Others were involved, others know more. Oneself, for various reasons, was at best a marginal figure. Exemplary for this is the following remark by Mrs./Mr. B.:

> *Nah. I didn't know anything. And then I always thought, oh, I should have known, why didn't anyone tell me anything. Of course I'm somewhat distanced from the Heidelberg rumor mill, that's why I'm sitting here. And an apartment in [town], that's quite impossible, so I'm not really into that.*

In addition, the reference to not wanting to be concerned with the private life of the head of the institute or other colleagues was a frequently mentioned argument for being uninvolved. Many interviewees also claimed that they were outside the "Heidelberg rumour mill" or outside the immediate institute scene. Many colleagues in training or in private practice worked at the Institute, but enjoyed the physical distance between their place of training or work on the one hand and their place of residence on the other. At the same time, this figure of reasoning also shows the distance that could be taken to the incidents, to the boundary violations and assaults, and ultimately to H. M. himself, or that can now be taken in the interview – as in the following quotation from Ms./Mr. C.:

> *Then I said, firstly (...) and secondly, I didn't want to know if they said, oh, he's started something with the colleague, I don't want to know that. I don't want to judge or evaluate or interfere, because that's a bunch of young people, and there's always some kind of ferment.*

The reference to respect for privacy and to the fact that these were encounters between adults is also found in many of the interviewees. Even if one might find some things disconcerting, subjectively there were no sufficient reasons for interfering. Ms./Mr. C. remembers H. M.:

> *I had thought they'd get it together somehow. And this (...) is more of a private oddity, a man who women (...) who is looking for.*

And:

> *Anyway, I noticed that he was there – and at some point it kind of turned up that there was a woman in [town] who had a child by him. So it became a bit too much.*

> *And then this story came up at the end of his work, with the young woman he then married, who I didn't even know was a patient. I thought he had met her somehow. Later it was said that she was (...), she was then assessed, whether he treated her, I don't know. Anyway, he got her pregnant and then they got married.*

Similarly, Mrs./Mr. A.:

> *So I mean, so the accusations weren't about the young [patient] at all. After they got married, as far as I could hear from my [place], this topic was over. And then – but now don't ask me how – the accusations arose that he had been so intensive with the boys during these delegation assessments (...). So these are the things that I then found out afterwards.*

The forms of dependency described above are not only evident in H. M.'s small gestures of accommodation, but above all in the structure of the institute. H. M. was not only the director of the institute, but at the same time also the chairman of the board, which ultimately meant that he acted as a supervisory body of himself. Thus, there were repeated demands on the part of the members for more financial transparency. Questions were asked as to where certain funds were going. A candidate for training at the time remarked:

No one can name exactly who was on the board when H. M. was head of the institute.

However, many interviewees, including two of the interviewees focused on here, remember that the general meetings during H. M.'s time, but also beyond, were incredibly boring, as many things were not discussed or could not be addressed. Ms./Mr. B. said:

And there was M. P., who was also only a pro forma pre-(…), I don't know exactly, I don't know any internals. I was rarely there. But I know from this older colleague that there were four people sitting around. They served their time and that was it. And done.

Mrs./Mr. C's recollections point in a similar direction:

Those are meetings like that, two or three people came. It was quite strange, it wasn't like in any other institution that a larger number come or feel responsible, but it was so, yes, strange.

Another peculiarity, from which a specific dependence arose, is the personal union of doctor, institute and training director. This meant that all patients (children and adolescents) who were treated as part of a training case had to be seen and diagnosed by H. M. and given an indication. If one had opposed him as a training candidate or had conflicts with him, a continuation of the training would have been difficult, if not impossible, at least with regard to the treatment of training cases. Thus the head of the institute had a special position of power, which was only rectified after the disclosure in 1993 in favour of a division into several persons with corresponding functions. Ms./Mr. B.:

Mr. H. M. was the director of the institute and for a long time also on the board of directors or chairman of the board. We then changed that afterwards, we always said in the statutes that we now separate the fact that there is a managing director and a board of directors. That was, for example, one of the consequences of that.

Similarly, Mrs./Mr. A.:

After H. M. left, the institute was reorganized. H. M. was the sole ruler. He was the head of training, he was the head of the institute, he was all sorts of things.

The position of the 'autocrat' was further underpinned by his training as a medical doctor and analytical child and adolescent psychotherapist and psychoanalyst for adults, as can be seen from Mrs./Mr. C's statements:

> *Normally the child therapists, those who finished, can't become teaching analysts at all, for whatever reason, they need the adult teaching analysts. H. M. was an exception, because he (...) was a medical doctor and analyst, the others are usually social professions.*

But H. M. did not only know how to use his function as head of the institute, he also made himself and the institute indispensable as a data supplier for scientific studies. Even after leaving the institute, H. M. contributed to the reputation of AKJP-Heidelberg. Regardless of the fact that his cooperation partners judge their cooperation with him in retrospect as "probably very clumsy", these activities were not insignificant for the existence of the Institute in times of recognition of guideline psychotherapy procedures.

To substantiate the impression that the interviewees described in more detail here tended a priori to perceive themselves in the position of the attacked, the following passage from the interview with Ms./Mr. C. also fits:

> *And then I thought, maybe we're from the wrong school or the wrong church or wrong direction, we're not orthodox analysts, we're other analysts, so where the forefathers were allowed to work in the Nazi era, so to speak, and were not persecuted, not really persecuted, but (...)?*

For the interviewee (but also for some other interview partners), the "persecution" of the Children's Institute does not begin with the accusations against H. M., but is already located in the prehistory of the Institute. This begins with the confrontation with the former Göring Institute and later AOK Institute under Dührssen's leadership, in which H. M. was active as head of the Children's Institute. The pattern of "feeling attacked", which is historically founded in this way, of behaving as if in an interrogation and entrenching oneself in a defensive position, prevents a differentiated, dialogically oriented discussion of certain events, so that difficult feelings are also produced in the countertransference.

While Ms./Mr. A. and Ms./Mr. C. maintain this style of resistance throughout the interview, the opportunity for self-reflexive reflection opens up for Ms./Mr. B. in the course of the interview:

> *And what he has now with her, what she has in this H. M. story – and then I thought, obviously with all of us – there are quite strange defensive attitudes or reproachful attitudes or whatever. So she, to my mind, has nothing to do with it at all. But please. I don't know. Yes. So.*

And then:

A: Well, but what concerns me most was this, how is it that one is so stuck in a certain attitude. And you should have gotten over that. Even -
I: That you were in your attitude -
A: Yes.
I: – stuck -
A: Yes.
I: In what way?
A: Well, always the same thinking and not getting anywhere there.
I: After that became known.
A: After it was all done. Until today, and nothing has changed.
I: What do you mean there, stuck in attitude?
A: Yeah, yeah, I mean this, this, uh, feeling so attacked.
[crying]. Nobody attacks you there, I don't know.
I: As a person or as a representative of AKJP (Heidelberg)?
A: Both. Certainly I'm very – that's what I thought then last summer, I'm very identified with this institute. Yes. Because I've been there for so long. And I'm also so committed to it, where of course a lot of things annoy me. Of course. I thought it's strange that you always think the same. You don't usually do that. You always get a bit further by thinking things. And then I always think, I said to [my partner], that can't be true, that it haunts me endlessly. That is a strange sign, that shows that something is virulent. Today we would say it's a trauma story or something. And of course there was also a split in the institute. So it is certainly not the case that there was only a split between the IPP (Heidelberg – Mannheim) and the AKJP (Heidelberg), but certainly also within the institute.

Ms./Mr. B. identifies her/his highly charged affectivity, which repeatedly appears in the subject matter, as an indication of traumatic material. This does not find language, but is expressed exclusively in affect. Emotions are expressed without inner regulation. Even if the narrator knows that this is irrational, he/she cannot react otherwise at first. It is not possible to find a long desired calming down, because – as is known from psychotherapy – the non-digested in the sense of a lack of verbalization comes up again and again (Bion 1991). Metaphorically, so to speak, we can speak here of the necessity of "metabolizing" in that the undigested must be chewed through in order to be able to swallow it (Bion 2013). In reading our interview transcripts, this process also manifests itself more frequently in countertransference: The more the actors try to convey calm and distance, the more affect-laden one becomes in the countertransference. This also explains the heated atmosphere during the decision on the commission for the scientific inquiry of the "Causa H. M." in the context of the general meetings in 2018. The atmosphere reported in this context depicted what had not been processed. According to Kernberg, splits as defense mechanisms always emerge when "idealized" and "pursuing" parts could not be integrated in the object relationship (Kernberg and Strauß

2001). But to all appearances not only this integration is missing, but it is furthermore noticeable that one's own role and one's own parts are little reflected in some interviews, so that the style of defense often cannot be abandoned. One feels reminded of two camps, both struggling for (emotional and cognitive) understanding of their situation.

We have described above how mutual accusations of guilt repeatedly lead to the ignition of affective breakthroughs and correspondingly violent conflicts. In the sense of a sustainable inquiry of the "Causa H. M." for the AKJP Institute Heidelberg, it seems important to us that the backgrounds of the feelings identified and described here are subjected to a reflexive consideration and negotiated on a linguistic level. In this sense, the considerations of Mrs./Mr. B. in the last quotation could function as a model.

Theoretical Models: Individual and Institutional Victimization of Sexual Violence

8

8.1 Abuse System – Disclosure System – Help System

We have developed a background heuristic that is able to contribute to the understanding of what happened in connection with the sexual boundary violations and sexual abuse of power by H. M. on the basis of the analysis of disclosure trajectories after sexual abuse (Mosser, 2009). By distinguishing between the abuse system, the disclosure system and the help system, this empirically based model offers the possibility of a fundamental location of the complex dynamics that are grouped around sexual violence.

Our analyses have shown that such dynamics follow certain phase progressions:

> *These are characterized by newly forming system configurations with different affiliations in each case. These emerge in the wake of critical transitional events. Distinctive systems, i.e. systems that are very specific and clearly distinguishable from other social environments, form as a result of the sexual abuse (abuse system), as a result of the disclosure (disclosure system) and as a result of the efforts to obtain professional support (help system).* (Mosser, 2009, p. 155)

In the following, it will be shown that this model has a certain explanatory potential for the pronounced resistance to disclosure with regard to H. M.'s acts against girls, boys and women. The analysis in this regard is based on a retrospective description of distinguishable system configurations in certain phases of the violent events and the discursive handling of them.

P. Caspari et al., *At some point there has to be peace and quiet!*,
https://doi.org/10.1007/978-3-658-39785-2_8

Abuse System

The first step is an analysis of various abuse systems that were constituted within the framework of the extraordinarily heterogeneous crime patterns in which H. M. entangled various groups of people. First of all, it is important to note here that every sexual boundary violation constitutes a system of abuse. Especially for the constellations of crimes in the case of H. M., it is paradigmatically true that the sexual acts establish an exclusive social space, which is essentially supported by two pillars: Pressure for secrecy, power of interpretation of the perpetrator. Every boy who had to undress in the examination room inevitably became part of such a configuration. The interpretive power of the pediatrician is inviolable: he constructs a situation in which the sexually toned act, by which the child patient is irritated, disturbed, and shamed, appears as a medically necessary intervention. Where the perpetrator's interpretive power finds such a reliable framework, the pressure for secrecy is reducible. On the one hand, the abuse system is exclusive because the whole subtle arrangement that the perpetrator groups around the sexualized act cannot be seen by any critical authority. On the other hand, it bears traits of a superficial transparency: description of investigation techniques in protocols with the aid of a diffuse psychoanalytical diction: extension of the power of interpretation into the partially public space of the institute. The cooperation of the victims is weak in these systems of abuse: On the one hand, the one-time encounter in the context of a second sight enables a silent escape, on the other hand, some children refuse further appointments with H. M.. We know nothing of increasingly massive sexual abuse acts towards children in the course of longer therapy processes. We only have knowledge of being forced to undress, of "evaluations" of the children, of touching of the penis, of shaming questions. These systems of abuse seem rather short-term, but are nevertheless potentially traumatizing.

Those configurations of violence in which young women are entangled by the psychotherapist H. M. in the course of therapies have a different structure. It should be noted that the abuse system is already formed through assaultive glances, insinuating remarks and irritating touching, which H. M. practiced not infrequently in the first therapy session. The exclusivity of the relationship is created by the structure of the psychotherapeutic setting and the unchallenged power of interpretation of the perpetrator: He "knows" that it allegedly helps young women if he intrusively questions them about sexual violence experiences they have suffered in the past or if such experiences are "reenacted". He can act out the belief that it helps the young woman if he, the therapist, "replaces" the young man from whom she has been so bitterly disappointed. Such a system of abuse is solidified by the increasingly offensive sexualization of the psychotherapeutic setting. The compulsion to secrecy need no longer be the consequence of explicit threats from the abuser; it is internalized by the young women victim as a logical imperative: shame about the sexual in psychotherapy. Guilt for having become increasingly involved (cf. Wilson et al., 2006). A clandestine dyadic space develops that functions according to its own laws, namely the laws of the psychotherapist endowed with an excess of power (Krutzenbichler, 1998). From this perspective, no further explanation is needed on the question of whether such a system of abuse persists after psychotherapy has ended. In the cases known to us, R. R. and E. M., clearly describable abuse systems had undoubtedly been established at the time of the termination of therapy, within the framework of which the further developments are to be located.

Superficially more complicated appears the attribution of H. M.'s relationships with adult training candidates and teaching analysands to the structural logic of abuse systems. The retrospective view, however, allows unmistakable insights: Exclusive space of the psychotherapeutic setting, abuse of power, offensive sexualization, pathological suffering of the women affected (cf. Hirsch, 2012; Schleu et al., 2018). Again, the problem of interpretive power, which per se plays a problematic role in the psychoanalytic method and takes the relentless path of derailment via the active sexualization of the therapeutic relationship. Abuse systems are characterized by being denied as such by the perpetrator and inaccurately classified as such by the victims. This too expresses the unequal distribution of power. It is important to note that the systems of abuse in which trainee analysts became entangled were subject to a relatively low degree of coercion to maintain secrecy, because the perpetrator's power of interpretation went beyond the exclusivity of the two-way relationship: a private matter between two adults.

Disclosure System

A consideration of disclosure systems sharpens the contours of the abuse systems to which they refer. According to our analyses, disclosure systems are characterized by the fact that they constitute a social space of belonging that is significant for the victim, within which ambivalences, fears, cognitive processes and ethical evaluations are given a reliable emotional framework. Since the disclosure of sexual violence is usually associated with psychological stress on the part of the victim, we speak of so-called "disclosure crises", which are usually accompanied by strong fears and uncertainties. In such critical transitional phases, "crisis dyads" prove to be the structure that – as a reactualization of early attachment representations – seems particularly suitable for coping with such stressful transitional experiences. A simple form of crisis dyad can be observed when the boy studied by H. M. tells his mother that he had to strip naked and that the doctor was looking at his penis. Through this communication, the potential for a system of disclosure is exposed that is clustered around the sexual assault. What is crucial at this point is how the mother responds. Indeed, the disclosure system is not defined by the boy's communication alone, but requires a social event in which disclosure is recognized as such. At this point, it is important to note that the development of disclosure systems is not necessarily accompanied by the dissolution of abuse systems. Initially, only a social and communicative frame of reference is formed that is distinguishable from the abuse system. Ideally, parents have taken their children's communications seriously and have not exposed them to further danger from contact with H. M.. Beyond this ideal case, it can be assumed that the second sifter's abuse systems often dissolved by the sheer fact that no further appointments were necessary, rather than by the fact that disclosure systems were configured. In individual cases that have come to our attention, disclosure systems developed with an enormous time lag, for example, in that affected children did not confide in their parents until they were adolescents, or in that case in which a criminal investigation is initiated almost 20 years late. Of particular importance here are those cases in which the AKJP-Heidelberg – especially in the mid/late 1990s – became aware of several cases of sexual boundary violations by H. M. against children.

In this way, employees of the Institute became part of system configurations that could have become effective in the sense of disclosure systems. Corresponding social configurations receive their specific contours when they are thought of from the perspective of the victims: The question is: What does it mean for the (former) child when a therapist tells an employee of the institute that she was informed by parents that their child had suffered sexual boundary violations in an examination situation at H. M.? And: What responsibility arises from this for persons and institutions who are "invited" in this way, as it were, to act as part of a system of disclosure? It can be said that such "invitations" were regularly rejected by AKJP-Heidelberg and its staff. It was not understood that it is not only about collecting information, but also about the needs of the affected child and the disclosure system that had already grouped around this child: Which decisions should the communicating therapist make? What pressures are the child's parents facing? It is important to understand that disclosure systems only have a "private" character in the shape of the crisis dyad, whereas they are very often formed from institutional instances: Youth Welfare Office, police, youth welfare institutions, specialized counselling centres, schools, etc. This institutional involvement naturally results in institutional responsibility. It can therefore be said with regard to affected children (and also adolescents) that the psychotherapeutic institutes involved have regularly warded off the possibility of becoming parts of disclosure systems.

With regard to the configuration of disclosure systems for sexual boundary violations against young adult female patients, statements can only be made about

R. R. and E. M. With regard to other victims, however, it can be stated that no institutional disclosure systems were formed that would have been suitable to initiate criminal and/or professional consequences for the perpetrator. It is not possible to assess to what extent there have been communications in the private sphere or in therapeutic settings. The cases R. R. and E. M., on the other hand, must be seen as examples of the development of dysfunctional disclosure systems. In both cases there was an institutional discourse which problematized the relationship of the young women with the psychotherapist H. M., who was decades older, and explicitly considered it from the point of view of sexual exploitation: the youth welfare office, the police and the two training institutes IPP-Heidelberg-Mannheim and AKJP-Heidelberg dealt with the two cases within the framework of their respective different professional mandates, but no disclosure system was formed over decades which would have been suitable to dissolve permanently stable abuse systems. The findings are clear: the abuse systems initiated by the psychotherapist proved to be completely robust against the challenges of a potentially quite powerful institutional arrangement that dealt with the cases.

No dyadic constellations could develop in which the ambivalences and fears of the young women affected could have been resolved in the sense described above. Nothing could compete with the existential dependence on the perpetrator, which was cemented both by the shared children and by the glaring imbalance in terms of social and material resources between the young mothers and the psychotherapist. A striking indication of the reliable existence of these abuse systems can be seen in the fact that the young women apparently did not make any statements to the institutions that would have been suitable for initiating functioning disclosure systems. The victims were still trapped in the perpetrator's system of secrecy and manipulation. They could not express that they had already suffered sexual assaults by H. M. during the therapeutic treatment. A marriage between perpetrator and victim does not defuse an abuse system but perpetuates it. At this point, at the latest, it can be said that individual members of the AKJP Institute Heidelberg, by "blessing" a marriage resulting from an abuse system with their benevolent presence, themselves became part of the abuse system. It would have been their responsibility to form a disclosure system together with other institutions that would have enabled the young woman to escape a permanently damaging relationship constellation. In this way, however, the perpetrator's power of interpretation, complete dependence and sexual exploitation remained.

The systems of abuse in which female teaching analysts and training candidates became entangled only acquired their clearly recognizable contours through the formation of functional systems of disclosure. Prior to this, the social systems that clustered around the relationships between the women and H. M. were contaminated by the perpetrator's interpretive power. The principle of secrecy was only applied with limited consistency: joint trips, pictures in the institute, open communication about the relationship. The fact that (almost) all the women affected were married seemed to be rather conducive to the social establishment of their relationship with H. M., because those who were outraged about it might have attracted the reproach of "philistinism". One did not want to take offence at the air of illegitimacy that clung to the relationships of the head of the institute with female candidates for training. Ideas of sexual violence, sexual exploitation, rape or sexual abuse did not seem to apply to the partially opaque events between H. M. and training candidates and teaching analysts, which took place before the eyes of the institute's public. For a long time, therefore, no systems of disclosure could develop. As far as can be reconstructed, everything suddenly changed at the end of 1992: complete collapse of the perpetrator's power of interpretation. Whatever led to the fact that suddenly several women turned to the director of the IPP-Heidelberg-Mannheim and scandalized H. M.'s boundary violations in the context of teaching analyses: At this point a classical system of disclosure was constituted, which – as far as we can gather from the available data – was connected with a lasting dissolution of the respective abuse systems. Presumably, emotionally charged crisis dyads formed in therapeutic settings (possibly including communication with the IPP-Heidelberg-Mannheim executive) that enabled the women to persevere through their undoubtedly extremely stressful disclosure efforts. It is safe to assume that the processes involved were accompanied by the painful realization of having been enmeshed in an abusive system – in some cases for many years. In contrast to the young female patients who had been impregnated by H. M., functional systems of disclosure (albeit only in the sense of system-immanent solutions) can be identified in the cases involving teaching analysands and training candidates. In this context, it is important to note that the functionality is not shown in the institutional handling of H. M., but in the protection of the affected women from the perpetrator: the systems of abuse in which they were entangled were dissolved, the perpetrator's power of interpretation was broken, and secrecy was placed where it seemed helpful to the victims.

Help System

The help system is different from the disclosure system. While the social formation of the disclosure system primarily serves to dissolve the structure of the abuse system, which is determined by secrecy and power imbalances, the help system primarily refers to coping with the consequences on the part of the victims. A special feature in the constellation examined here is that there is initially a far-reaching overlap between the help system and the abuse system: this applies to all those children, adolescents and young women who were referred to H. M. for an examination or therapy on the basis of a possible psychotherapeutic indication and were shamed, touched and sexually exploited there. The doctor and psychotherapist was visited in his function as a representative of the help system. However, he often transformed this into an exclusive system of abuse. The form of help system discussed here relates specifically to coping with the consequences that the experiences within the abuse system entailed. We know little about the extent to which child patients addressed the abuse by the doctor after their contact with H. M. in the context of subsequent help. This does not seem improbable, especially in the context of medical delegation to psychotherapists, since these patients came to psychotherapeutic treatment after their contact with H. M. However, we do not have any information from psychotherapists according to which child patients would have expressed themselves about H. M.'s irritating examination practices in the context of therapy. (For understandable reasons this does not mean that there were no such reports). At least in one case we know that a pre-adolescent girl affected by sexual boundary violations had to struggle with severe psychological stress as a result of the examination situation. She developed strong fears towards male doctors and therefore avoided any contact with medical-therapeutic help. Only after many years did she feel able to address H. M.'s assaults in the context of psychotherapy. The data available to us do not allow a generalization of this episode. Further above, it was noted that individual children turned to their parents with the communication about H. M.'s shameful examination practices. In no case is it known that such revelations gave rise to determined processes of seeking help. As a rule, these children were in psychotherapy for other reasons, whereby nothing can be said about the extent to which these contributed to coping with this disturbing experience.

Overall, it can be assumed that the majority of those who were sexually exploited by H. M. had a certain affinity to the psychotherapeutic help system. Particularly in the case of the adolescent and adult patients, the question therefore arises as to how and to what extent the victims expressed their stressful experiences with H. M. to their later psychotherapists. Furthermore, it is unclear to what extent the psychotherapists addressed with such messages actually constituted help systems in the sense of overcoming these experiences. We know from E. M. that she apparently visited several psychotherapists in the course of her marriage, whereby the effect of the help system had to remain limited in view of the fact that she had been under the direct influence of the abuse system for several decades. The same can be assumed of R. R., since a clear demarcation from the abuse system controlled by H. M. is not recognizable. In the case of those women who turned to the head of the IPP-Heidelberg-Mannheim in 1992/1993, successful transitions into the help system can be assumed. By supporting them in their disclosure, the possibility was opened to develop changed, albeit painful, perspectives on their experiences with H. M., which they were very likely to be able to establish permanently in the context of psychotherapies.

In the overall view, the sequence abuse system – disclosure system – help system presents itself as fragile in most of the cases that refer to sexual exploitation by H. M.. We find a large number of unactivated disclosure potentials in the sense that disclosure systems either did not constitute themselves at all or turned out to be ineffective or even dysfunctional. In many cases, a pronounced permanence of the abuse systems set up by H. M. must be stated, which seems shocking in view of the severe psychological damage that was associated with it for the victims. The case of the young patient, whose marriage to H. M. perpetuated the abuse system undisturbed in front of the eyes of various disclosure systems, is particularly impressive. A large number of people have been harmed by H. M.'s actions. Unfortunately, we can say little about how many of them received the help that enabled them to cope with these experiences in a stable manner. It is well known that such help does not necessarily take the form of psychotherapy. Healing private relationships, counseling, social supports, or self-help initiatives can be equally effective help (Helming et al., 2011). At the very least, our data allow us to assume that the victims, their parents, or others who knew about it communicated H. M.'s sexual boundary violations to the psychotherapy scene in and around Heidelberg in multiple ways. The extent to which this scene proved to be a functioning help system cannot be assessed here. However, it is clearly recognizable that the revelations made behind the walls of the treatment rooms mostly remained there: Isolated, disconnected strands of disclosure. The extent to which the psychotherapist bound to secrecy is necessarily prevented from becoming part of a system of disclosure, or is prevented from becoming part of it, must be the subject of further discussion.

8.2 Latent Processes and Manifest Index Events

In the course of our research on sexual violence and child maltreatment in institutional contexts, we have identified – starting from a lifespan perspective – certain biographical processes that significantly modulate the coping experience of victims (Mosser, 2019; Mosser & Hackenschmied, 2018). In this regard, we have identified four central aspects, namely (1) awareness, (2) remembrance, (3) disclosure, and (4) seeking help, whereby the particular dynamic of these phenomena is that they do not follow a linear movement towards resolution or dissolution, but rather that there is a sequence of latent processes and certain index events, often spanning decades, in the course of which the earlier experience is reenacted in a temporally overformed manner. The following quote from an interviewee precisely illustrates this dynamic: "The funny thing is that it always starts to appear like this, then it disappears again. It appears so eruptively, once like this, huh, somehow like this. Then it collapses again."

What is important here is that both processes and index events take place against the background of changing social conditions and discourses.

The "Causa H. M." stimulates reflection on the extent to which this conception, originally developed for individuals, could also be applied to definable institutional systems. Since we have a variety of data available, especially on the "course of coping" of the AKJP-Heidelberg, it seems useful to outline the sequence of latent processes and manifest index events for this institute in order to generate findings with explanatory value.

Awareness

Awareness is one of the central mechanisms in coping with sexual violence suffered (Draucker & Martsolf, 2008; Harvey et al., 1991; Rieske et al., 2018). Becoming aware means acquiring an internal conception of what has happened that has the inherent potential for healing. Moreover, becoming aware is a process that relies on interpersonal discourse and social validation. It is known from research that it takes a certain amount of cognitive and moral development to form an increasingly consistent, socially validatable, and intrapsychically processible picture of sexual violence suffered (Draucker & Martsolf, 2008; Orbuch et al., 1994). As described above, sexual violence is subject to the perpetrator's power of interpretation. Becoming aware therefore means: questioning these interpretations, emancipating oneself from the perpetrator's constructions of reality within the exclusive space of the abuse system, developing one's own reliable concepts about what happened (Mosser, 2020; Unabhängige Aufarbeitungskommission, 2017, 2019a). One can ask: How did the process of becoming aware of the AKJP Institute Heidelberg take shape? It can be stated that as long as H. M. functioned as the head of the institute, there was no even remotely stable awareness within the AKJP-Heidelberg regarding the damage that H. M. inflicted on other people (female colleagues, young adult patients, girls and boys) under abuse of his power. After all, this must be asserted for a period of 18 years. As far as can be seen, no interpretations of his behaviour were virulent which could have been formulated in terms of "abuse", "violence" or "exploitation". It can therefore be assumed that the institutional level of awareness corresponded for a long time to that of people who are entangled in an abuse system and exposed to the manipulations of the perpetrator without protection. Retrospectively, this is proven, among other things, by the remarkable formulation already quoted above from the letter of the members of the VAKJP Nordbaden in 1993, who overlooked the "atmosphere of boundary transgressions" or "accepted them with ironic commentary". As different as the ethical or emotional feelings may have been in relation to the more or less explicit behaviour of the head of the institute, an overall lack of institutional awareness of the associated dangers can be described as quite homogeneous. This is also expressed in the following interview sequence with a psychotherapist:

> *I: But that is, so relations between lecturers and training candidates was now, which quite occurred -*
> *A: Yes.*
> *I: And has that been addressed in any way or talked about?*
> *A: No.*

Against this background, the disclosures in 1993 form a clearly contoured index event, in the course of which significant processes of awareness were stimulated. For many, forebodings, feelings and hitherto insufficiently reflected perceptions combined to form a shape that enabled a changed evaluation of H. M.'s behaviour. Since the information about the pregnancy of the young (ex-)patient and the transgressions of boundaries towards training analysands also triggered a high degree of insecurity and threat, the potential for possible processes of becoming conscious was, however, also averted by many people. The clash of forced and defended processes of consciousness-raising ultimately created the strongly pronounced image of an institutional split in consciousness, which determined the further course of coping at AKJP-Heidelberg to a great extent (cf. Burka et al., 2019). One interviewee brings this to the point in the following concise way:

> *They all knew very different things.*

In the following years, the movement of the collective consciousness of the Institute was not linear and discontinuous. Interesting is the accumulation of index events between 1993 and 2000: conferences, messages from therapists, complaints from parents and finally the group "Past – Present – Future". It can be said that the AKJP-Heidelberg was repeatedly confronted with offers of awareness which the institution as a whole was unable to process constructively. By no means does the picture present itself of a homogeneous repression of the events surrounding H. M., but rather of a psychological and social dynamic in which selective, occasion-related processes of awareness of individual protagonists of the institute could not form an organizational event. Metaphorically, one could speak here of the structure of a trauma consciousness: Isolated, encapsulated psychological processes that do not find access to the "ego control" of the institution. Despite various incentives from the outside and despite various efforts of significant members of the institute, the "collective consciousness" of AKJP-Heidelberg remains fragmented. Individual examples show that even significant individual processes of becoming conscious, which are connected with fundamental re-evaluations of earlier experiences, do not contribute to the integration of the fragmented structure of the institute's consciousness. As a result, the picture that emerges is one of institutional consciousness paralysis beginning in the early 2000s and continuing, with the exception of minor movements, until about 2016. Retrospectively, the impression arises of a pronounced latency period, in which the AKJP-Heidelberg apparently considers the "long past" history as "processed". This can certainly be understood in analogy to individual processing after experiences of violence, in the course of which phases of "completed awareness" can be observed, which allow a relatively increased functionality in coping with life. After this latency period, a series of significant index events occur from 2016 onwards, which lead to a massive reactivation of streams of consciousness: The seminar of the institute's director and ethics officer, the criminal complaint against H. M. from the family, the court case, the "ZEIT" article, and the founding of an inquiry group that was internal of the institute. These events interrogate the Institute's past and make possible an awareness that is not obscured by the pressing demands of a threatening present (as in 1993). But although the temporal distance allows for a higher degree of reflection, the fragmented structure of the institutional consciousness becomes recognizable again, because massive questionings of inquiry processes still exist, as they emerge from the assessment of one interviewed psychotherapist:

> *I thought that someone somewhere had nothing else to do and thought he had to do something important by pricking a blister somewhere again, which in my opinion had actually been squeezed out as a pus bag for a long time (…). Where I did not get why now, after everything was actually eaten off, why does it reappear now. So I have no explanation for it.*

And yet the movement of discourses now seems much more integrative than in earlier times. This certainly implies the occurrence of fierce conflicts mainly due to mutual recriminations, but the process of becoming aware now seems to be forming into an institutional happening. There are younger members of AKJP-Heidelberg who are questioning the Institute about its past and there are older members who are ready to give answers. In seminars, general meetings and inqury groups, places of discourse seem to be forming that are not contaminated by the attempt of interest-bound obfuscation, but seem to express an actual interest in what happened in the past and in the consequences to be drawn from it for the future. This movement is not homogeneous, but collective processes of awareness are not characterized by their homogeneity, but by the willingness to engage in conflictual discourse and the attempt to develop a narrative that can function as a socially accepted reference for the future – in this case: of AKJP-Heidelberg (Burka et al., 2019; Mosser et al., 2018; Unabhängige Aufarbeitungskommission, 2019b).

Remembering/Forgetting

It is important to distinguish remembering from awareness. While awareness refers to a change in the hermeneutic framework in relation to certain events, remembering is solely concerned with their representation in memory. The problem of remembering after traumatic events, and particularly in relation to suffering sexual violence, has been extensively described in the literature (Kavemann et al. 2015a; McNally, 2005). Remembering and forgetting fulfil significant functions here in the psychological coping with what has been experienced. In this context, it should be pointed out, among other things, that traumatic amnesia should certainly not be seen solely as a consequence of a biological survival reaction in the context of the acute phase of the experience of stress, but that memory representations of sexual violent experiences are often much more strongly shaped by motivational, ethical and social processes. Not remembering represents not only a function of denial or repression, but also of trivialization or re-evaluation. A collective discourse about sexual violence is often grouped around the individual representation of memory, which is accompanied by attributions of meaning, scandalizations and/or trivializations. In this respect, remembering and forgetting are by no means independent of the processes of awareness described above, but they are something fundamentally different from these processes of awareness. Transferred to the analyses carried out here, the question now arises as to what was represented in the collective memory of the AKJP-Heidelberg over all these years and not so much how these memory representations were interpreted. First of all, it can be clearly demonstrated that institutional memory does not function additively any more than individual memory (cf. Welzer, 2002). However, it is also interesting to note that the Institute's efforts to develop a collective additive memory representation of the events surrounding H. M. were conspicuously weak. The impression arises that corresponding initiatives were only repeatedly initiated by the Institute's ethics officer, although they were unable to contribute to the development of a collective memory due to the lack of resonance on the part of the Institute's public. The overall picture is once again one of latent remembering/forgetting, which has been irritated by significant "memory events" but not sustainably expanded.

It is important that the remembering already began long before 1992/1993: memories of "sultry" institute parties where bare-breasted dancing on tables took place, memories of fellow students who told of their intimate relationship with H. M., memories of communications that H. M. slept with female patients, memories of the former patient whose common child with H. M. appeared again and again at the AKJP-Heidelberg, memories through photos that were publicly accessible at the institute, etc.. The history of AKJP-Heidelberg and IPP-Heidelberg-Mannheim was full of memories of boundary transgressions by H. M. even before 1992/1993, especially since the list started here has a purely exemplary character and does not come close to expressing the extent of the talk about "ambiguous" behavior by H. M.. What is special about it is that it was in the nature of these manifold individual memories not to be able to unite into a collective memory. We have seen above how a multitude of potential threads of disclosure came to nothing because there was a pronounced disconnectedness with regard to the perception of conspicuousness in H. M.'s behavior. Because talk was not given a chance to coalesce into a systematic discourse, individual memory representations kept getting lost in the isolation of a consciousness that lacked social validation of its perceptions. Our interviews reveal that symptomatic flare-ups of memory were surrounded by an ocean of motivationally generated forgetting. One interviewee describes a phase of remembering and forgetting, which began with the fact that she/he had already become aware of H. M.'s meanwhile disclosed sexual boundary violationsin the Heidelberg psychotherapy scene before the beginning of her/his training at the AKJP-Heidelberg:

> *Yeah, I thought it was inappropriate, sure, I thought it was inappropriate. But then I forgot about it again. But now, of course, now I find it – so now I found it quite crass, I was also in the trial.*

For 18 years, both the AKJP-Heidelberg and the IPP-Heidelberg-Mannheim moved in this "amnesia-affine" atmosphere, since there obviously existed institutional framework conditions which, here as well as there, referred budding observations and memories back again and again into the isolated space of individual consciousness. This has the effect of the memory structure of a young abuse victim who, between shame, manipulation, disturbance, fear, silence, denial and repression, seeks a bearable path towards functionality. An important principle of protection here is to avoid memories.

Here, too, the events of 1992/1993 represent an index experience of the collective memory: One had just performed collective memory work in the context of the jubilee on the occasion of the 40th anniversary of the AKJP-Heidelberg and the 60th birthday of its director and had expressed oneself half amused, half irritated about the existence of H. M.'s one-year-old child with a young (ex-)patient, when the impulse for a completely different form of remembering was given from outside. In this way the structure of the fragmented memory of the AKJP-Heidelberg became completely manifest. Now the numerous, unconnected memories could have found a discursive place, but the institution as a whole proved robust to the threats exerted by multiple emerging strands of individual memory. Individual memory proved patchy, inconsistent, doubtful and weak. It may have found its way into supervisions, intervision, teaching analyses and psychotherapies, but it was not capable of establishing a conscious collective memory of the institution AKJP-Heidelberg that would have made the institute capable of acting. This also has to do with the specific characteristics of the psychotherapeutic situation as described by one of the psychotherapists we interviewed:

> *You know, that also has a lot to do with the fact that the analysis is something very secret, which should remain protected, but where of course the door is opened to assumptions and unclear things. It is – if an analysand claims that and that, then one does not know for a long time whether that is really the case. The respective analyst – but mostly it is men after all – can very largely retreat behind the fact that he does not have to make a statement. Or at least not in the institute.*

Like the memory of the abuse victim in the disclosure crisis, which investigators, prosecutors and judges work on again and again, the memory of the AKJP-Heidelberg in its disclosure crisis was surrounded by fears, doubts, ambivalences and threats. These dynamics prevented the necessary sorting of virulent memory contents, so that memory remained permanently fragile and fragmented. This structure also considerably restricted the possibility of integrating newly added information into the "institutional memory". Symptomatic of this is the handling of the numerous reports of sexual boundary violations by H. M. against children in the course of the 1990s. The impression is created that with each new piece of information that is added, already existing memories had to be "sacrificed". Never was all the information represented. Again and again it was "forgotten" that H. M. had impregnated two young female patients and that he had involved several training analysands in sexual relations. By the year 2000 at the latest, the "Past – Present – Future" group would have offered the possibility of integrating the sheer extent of the information available up to that time into an overall picture that should have led to appropriate consequences for evaluation and action. While even more information was generated through the analysis of old institute files, in other segments of the organization motivationally controlled forgetting apparently already set in again. Memories that could be rationalized individually could not be combined into a consistent collective memory even in the "inquiry group" in the year 2000, because it was apparently still not possible to cope with their extent. It seems as if – on an institutional level – every memory also revealed the necessity of forgetting. This corresponds to the ambivalence of the abuse victim, who tries to navigate biographically in the field of tension between the desire for processing and integration on the one hand and the fear of confrontation on the other. Forgetting plays a significant role in maintaining both individual and institutional functionality. With regard to AKJP-Heidelberg, the picture that emerges is of a collective of people who, in large numbers and for different reasons, are characterized by an individually motivated forgetting with regard to H. M.'s sexual boundary violations. This collective also includes individuals who are convinced of the necessity of remembering, but at the same time fail to transform individual memories into a collective institutional memory. From 2004 to 2016, the Institute (but not individuals among them also quite influential) appears by and large amnesic with respect to H. M. The inquiry seminar offered by the Institute's director and the ethics officer, the court case against H. M. and, in a special way, the appearance of the dossier in the "ZEIT" finally contribute to a serious reorganization of the Institute's memory. It becomes clear not only what was not known, but also the extent of what had been forgotten in the meantime. These are significant index events for the collective memory of the AKJP-Heidelberg. It also became clear that a written documentation of information accessible to all (in the form of the newspaper article) is an important tool for the development of an institutional memory. If you want to remember something, you write something down. What every child learns in school has been missed by the AKJP-Institute Heidelberg for decades. The most serious failure in this context is the failure to document the discourses in the "Past – Present – Future" group. If the institution does not document anything, the memories of the individuals are thrown back on their own memory organization. It may not be necessary to formulate written reference points for individual coping with experiences of victimization; however, an organization that forgoes reliable documentation when reflecting on its past is permanently thrown back on a disorganized sequence of latent memory processes and the emergence of intrusive memories.

Disclosure

Individual disclosure processes often follow a discontinuous pattern in which certain communications at different stages of life lead to the partial disclosure of the sexual violence suffered, although this is by no means always accompanied by a fundamental breaking of the secrecy imperative (Caspari, 2021a; Kavemann et al. 2015a; Rieske et al., 2018). An example are hints given by the child to parents that are not accurately understood by them or that do not lead to further behavioral consequences. Retrospectively, therefore, "disclosure biographies" can often be reconstructed, in which more or less sustained attempts at disclosure by victims can be identified, e.g. within the circle of friends, with relatives, in later partner relationships or in psychotherapy. "Disclosure" appears under this perspective not as a sharply contoured biographical experience, but as a selectively realized coping action under respectively changed biographical conditions (Mosser, 2019). The paradigmatic double character of disclosure as a latent process and manifest index event, which can be traced for individual biographies, is – as the example of AKJP-Heidelberg shows – also suitable for a transfer to institutional systems. We have seen above how a multitude of disclosure potentials or more or less dysfunctional uncovering systems were grouped around the deeds of the head of the institute H. M. The attempt to integrate these social events into an overall picture opens up a view of the pattern that is so typical of individual processes: a sequence of silences and individual manifest episodes of disclosure, which in a certain sense remain "unfinished" and therefore entail further disclosure requirements in later biographical phases (Caspari, 2021a; Keupp et al., 2019).

AKJP-Heidelberg did not "uncover" for the first time as an organization, or – to put it more precisely – it felt compelled to deal with the uncoverings brought to the institute, until 18 years after the start of the boundary violations by its institute director. We have seen that this first institutional disclosure event is similar to the disclosure of a minor(s), which leads to the removal of the perpetrator, but does not ensure lasting protection from his/her influence. Clearly, the events in 1993 had the character of unfinished disclosure events. Subsequently, it became apparent that narratives of boundary transgressions and assaults do not necessarily form disclosure episodes. This resembles those communicative events in which the communications of affected women and men in private settings or even in psychotherapies are not understood in their extent and their overall context. Something is said and something is heard, but there is no socially validated reconstruction of what has happened. What is left is the sense that what has been disclosed has not been "real". Therefore, despite the large amount of information that was brought to AKJP-Heidelberg until the early 2000s, there could be no question of a collectively shared "sense of disclosure". Something remained incomplete, misunderstood, undone. Subsequently, the AKJP-Heidelberg appears immunized in the sense of a pronounced insensitivity to further disclosure initiatives. An institutional feeling seems to have established itself that it has disclosed "enough", although this always remains contestable and unstable. Finally, symptomatic is the widespread horrified astonishment in the extended institutional public about the extent of H. M.'s sexual boundary violations in the wake of the 2017 court hearing and the publication of the 2018 "ZEIT" article. The extent of this astonishment points to the extent of the incompleteness of the disclosure attempts initiated since 1993. It almost seems as if virtually nothing had been disclosed until then. It becomes clear that the event of disclosure is not simply exhausted in the communication of information, but that it is about the development of a consistent script that takes on an increasingly recognizable shape through retrospective analysis. The reactions to the "ZEIT" article also open up a view of both the failures of the past and the reflexive potential of temporal distance – precisely as expressed in the following lines from T. S. Eliot's "Four Quartets":

> *We've had the experience,*
> *but did not grasp the meaning,*
> *When you explore the meaning,*
> *the experience returns*
> *in altered form ...*

Beyond moral evaluations, it becomes clear that the "institutional biography of disclosure" of the AKJP-Heidelberg had a spiral or iterative course, as is typical for individual processes of disclosure: communications and findings spark off clearly different effects in different phases, different time intervals from the initial event, and in different social configurations. In this sense, disclosure never comes to an end, so that it could be that the events surrounding the institute director H. M. will affect the consciousness of the AKJP Institute Heidelberg again and again "in a changed form".

Utilization of Assistance

The fourth coping dimension that we have described in our concept, in addition to awareness, remembering and disclosure, is that of seeking help. The dual character of latent processuality and manifest action is immediately evident from a psychological perspective: there are explicit attempts to turn to counselling centres, clinics or established psychotherapists in order to deal with the consequences of the sexual violence suffered. And there is "implicit coping action", which unfolds exemplarily in supporting social relationships, in stimulating activities and interests or in successful educational or professional initiatives (Caspari et al., 2021; Helming et al., 2011; Mosser, 2019). The explicit use of professional help usually represents a biographical marker that can be clearly distinguished from everyday efforts to lead a successful life. This does not answer the question of what "actually" helps, but the use of help is usually preceded by important processes such as the realization of the need for help and the search for and finding of people who offer help. Even if they do not always run synchronously in terms of time, "utilization biographies" have a similar structure to "disclosure biographies": since different forms of help prove suitable and useful in different phases of life, new help potentials always open up at different times. In addition, it may be that stressful life events make the urgent character of a need for help that is already considered "settled" once again visible. From this point of view, analogies to the institutional management of "stressful events" suggest themselves: The question about the "utilization behavior" of the "damaged" AKJP-Institute Heidelberg points to the impression of a pronounced helplessness of the institution in connection with the transgressions and assaults of its director. Up to the year 1993 it is not at all recognizable that individuals or groups had turned to outside authorities with the at least preliminary assessment that one had a problem in the institution with the behaviour of the director. For a professional system whose meaning and identity – to put it briefly – consists in offering help, this omission seems remarkable. In any case, the barely developed help-seeking behaviour of the professional helpers raises a variety of questions. When the manifest crisis of AKJP-Heidelberg occurred in 1993, some help-seeking movements finally seemed to develop. On an individual level, according to our information, at least sporadically supervision or teaching analyses were used to get an orientation in this complex situation. On an institutional level, however, it can be noted that help-seeking movements were almost exclusively self-referential: General meetings, group meetings, seminars, and the wide field of more or less intense conflicts. The establishment of contact with the umbrella organization VAKJP can be seen as an exception, through which at least smaller parts of the Institute experienced a strengthening, which manifested itself, among other things, in the organization of a conference in Heidelberg in 1997. Otherwise, the help-seeking movements were disparate, as the institution itself was marked by diverging interests. The crisis of the institute, which threatened its existence, was superficially "mastered" by the appointment of the interim solution M. P. and the institute director L. Z., who was brought in from outside. After a caesura in 1994, the "operation" of AKJP-Heidelberg was resumed and continued to the present day. However, the established mode of functioning of the institute was very soon and repeatedly disturbed by symptoms of a still existing need for help: messages from parents and colleagues about sexual boundary violations by H. M. against children; the need for inquiry expressed on various occasions within the institute; the repeated reference by the IPP-Heidelberg-Mannheim that H. M. was still active in powerful functions (above all as an expert) and as a psychotherapist in private practice. Metaphorically speaking, the institution found itself in the field of tension so typical for stressed individuals between maintaining everyday functionality on the one hand and confrontation with the noticeable need for help on the other. In this context, the question always arises: does the use of help and the associated confrontation with painful feelings and insights impair our functioning in everyday life? The Institute opted for what might be called a "help-seeking compromise" by redirecting the variously expressed needs for inquiry into the group "Past –

Present – Future". One might say that this is a kind of self-help in a sense that tends to be dysfunctional. The realizsation that not only individuals but also institutions could usefully turn to someone outside in order to be able to bring their own problems to reflexive processing was apparently not so pronounced as, for example, to make use of external organizational consulting or organizational development. The insight that the Institute was still by no means in a position to help itself in the year 2000 seems only possible in retrospective analysis. In the course of the following years, the picture of a functional but irritable institution presents itself. And here, too, the analogy to an individual who manages his life in a successful way, but who is also accompanied by the feeling that it would be better not to look too closely at certain aspects of his biography. Against this background it seems symptomatic that in parts of the Institute's public it is regarded as a betrayal when the ethics officer supplies the "ZEIT" journalist with "incriminating material" from the Institute's past. At this point, at the latest, the old lines of conflict that had more or less latently pervaded the functioning institute over all the years break open unmistakably and in part with great vehemence. The now formulated need for external "help" in the form of a scientific inquiry is accompanied by corresponding ambivalences within the institute, as can be seen not only from the following quotation from an interviewed psychotherapist:

> *... we award this contract, this alone – the way this happens speaks to the fact that this is highly problematic. There's no reasonable conversation. There are immediate accusations, counter-accusations, one would love to lash out at the other. One would love to lash out at the other! Quite irrational!*

Metaphorically, the arguments against working through the past include those rationales that discourage the burdened individual from seeking professional help: Disruption of everyday functioning, damage to impeccable reputation by admitting a need for help, and-in some cases: Unjustifiable time and cost. Overall, the institutional help-seeking and utilization behavior of AKJP-Heidelberg appears ambitious and – given the functionality maintained over the decades – efficient. Without doubt, however, there is something that has not been sufficiently processed to date, which is probably due to the fact that one had neglected to allow a critical, systematic and process-oriented view from the outside in time.

8.3 Knowledge Base in Different Systems

A social science model developed by Rieske et al. (2018) on the basis of empirical studies of disclosure processes following sexual violence is highly suitable for approaching the question of the conditions that prevented an adequate handling of H. M. 's acts. The representation of different bodies of knowledge in different social formations functions as a central aspect of this model. Against the background of Bronfenbrenner's sociologically based division (Bronfenbrenner et al., 1981) into onto-, micro-, meso- and macrosystems, the existence or absence of different bodies of knowledge is recalled. The authors make a fundamental distinction between event knowledge, discourse knowledge and process/structural knowledge. Event knowledge refers to the knowledge of what happened (e.g. a certain form of sexual boundary violation); discourse knowledge refers to the prevailing patterns of perception of sexual violence in the respective social structure (e.g. the question of what is okay and what is not okay in the sexual sphere). Finally, process/structural knowledge is – in short – present when people know what they have to do when they become aware of a sexual violation or when the victims know about institutional help options.

An analysis of the events in the environment of the AKJP-Heidelberg in connection with the transgressions of the head of the institute H. M. enables a retrospective diagnosis of available knowledge and the effects of corresponding deficits. For reasons of clarity, a rough distinction is made here between four constellations of offences initiated by H. M., namely (1) sexual boundary violations against boys and girls in childhood in the context of second sights and psychotherapies, (2) sexual assaults against girls and boys in adolescence, also in the context of second sights and psychotherapies, (3) sexual relations with young women during and after their psychotherapeutic treatment by H. M., and (4) sexual relations with teaching analysands/training candidates.

Sexual Assault Against Boys and Girls in Childhood

The basis of any intervention after sexual violence is an at least partially developed knowledge of the event. One must know approximately what happened in order to be able to draw consequences. This statement is not trivial insofar as information about sexual acts is often only available in fragments. From the perspective of the victims, the problem of memory representation of such experiences plays a major role here, so that it is often difficult to fall back on consistent event knowledge. With regard to sexual boundary violations against child patients, very clearly contoured potentials for event knowledge can be identified again and again over the decades: Boys report to their mothers that they had to strip naked at H. M.'s. Mothers complain to their psychotherapists about the doctor's boundary violating examination methods, and a number of second sight records exist in which at least irritating-seeming examination situations are documented. These protocols were typed by the secretary and read by the treating psychotherapists. Regardless of the assumption that the information given here is only the "tip of the iceberg", it becomes clear that event knowledge was represented on different system levels: On the level of the ontosystem we find those children who felt ashamed, irritated and/ or distressed by the examination situation with H. M. and can still remember the at least unpleasant character of this scene later. The parents who became aware of these boundary violations have event knowledge at the level of the microsystem, i.e. the immediate social reference system of the boy or girl affected. However, event knowledge also becomes available within the mesosystem, namely when the parents (and later perhaps the victims themselves) turn to institutions (educational counselling centres, police, etc.) or established psychotherapists. Knowledge of events in relation to sexual assaults against children therefore also exists at the AKJP-Heidelberg: It is known there, for example, that H. M. was interested in the erection of boys who were presented to him, that he asked the boys about masturbation practices and that they had to undress with him. This knowledge varies in different segments of the institute and at different times and could, in principle, have given rise to critical enquiry and intervention action. At this point, however, the problem of the lack of discourse knowledge arises with great vehemence, which in the present case would refer to the question: What does the investigative repertoire of a psychotherapeutic physician consist of in the context of second views? Are physical examinations indicated on professional grounds? If so, how is this justified and within what professional framework? How is this justified to parents? In view of the following quotation from a psychotherapist interviewed by us, however, it cannot even be assumed that in the 1970s there was a generally available knowledge of the discourse according to which sexual acts by adults against children represented a problem requiring intervention:

> *Sexual assault on and with children did not exist in my mind.*

Does this make the question obsolete, under which conditions the medical examination situation makes it necessary for children to undress and thereby also expose their genitals? Retrospectively, the impression arises that there was no approximately distinct discourse knowledge on this question in the environment of the AKJP-Heidelberg. It seemed that there was simply no conception of the criteria according to which a medical examination carried out in the context of psychotherapy would make it possible, necessary or even impossible to transgress the boundaries of shame of the children examined. Was it H. M.'s grotesque private theories that seemingly legitimized such boundary violations, or was it simply assumed that it was somehow all right? It was not until the end of the 1990s or the beginning of the 2000s that it came to be judged, at least selectively, that H. M. had clearly exceeded his medical competence through his examination methods. However, the impression arises that this was made possible more by the now available knowledge about the person H. M. and less by a professionally founded and sufficiently discussed discourse knowledge about examination methods in the psychotherapeutic setting. As before, the exclusive situation in the medical examination room can be considered ethically underdefined, since the question of what is medically necessary is subject to the interpretive power of the doctor and not to the subjective feelings of the child being examined. At least it seems to have been possible for H. M. as late as 2013, in the context of a criminal complaint against him, to use the discourse figure of the medically necessary examination to avoid sanctioning his assaults against a boy. With regard to the boundary violations against boys and girls that have become known, an insufficiently developed process/structural knowledge on the part of the micro- and mesosystems surrounding the children affected must also be stated in the overall view. For decades, corresponding communications have either been ignored or merely taken note of. Knowledge about institutional procedures that would have led to protection and help for the affected children and to sanctioning of H. M.'s sexual boundary violations did not seem to be represented in the systems involved. In principle, indications of possible sexual boundary violations require well-coordinated intervention, which can include both recourse to official authorities (youth welfare office, investigating authorities) and counselling assistance (e.g. specialist counselling centers, educational counselling centers ...). In fact, however, the picture of a pronounced paralysis of action as a reaction to indications of sexual boundary violations against children in the context of the examinations by H. M. emerges. Such reports are "processed" self-referentially within the AKJP-Heidelberg, but according to our data there is no coordinated procedure involving external counselling instances. One learns in 1995 and 2013 of criminal charges against H. M. because of such assaults against children and apparently refrains from the attempt to take such index events as a reason for careful cooperation with the prosecuting authorities. It is not recognizable that the AKJP-Heidelberg would ever have had a plan on how to deal with the repeatedly emerging indications of such boundary violations. Due to the fact that H. M. was allowed to examine and treat children for many decades despite corresponding indications, it can be assumed that the parents of the children affected also lacked process/structural knowledge. The fact that the two criminal charges of which we are aware fizzled out ineffectively completes the picture of an uncoordinated, haphazard reaction pattern on the part of the adults gathered in the various micro- and mesosystems in the environment of the children affected, which was characterized by gaps in knowledge. This also includes information about the ineffectiveness of corresponding structures at AKJP-Heidelberg.

Sexual Boundary Violations Especially Against Adolescent Girls

With regard to sexual assaults, especially on female youths, there is – as far as we know – no usable knowledge of events over decades. That there were such incidents is proven by examples 4, 5 and 8 described in Sect. 4.1. Consequently, no well-founded assumptions can be made about what discourse knowledge would have been drawn upon in the 1970s and 1980s, when it was learned that the psychotherapist H. M. grabbed adolescent girls' breasts, asked them about their masturbation practices, offered them to try out sexual acts together or to "reenact" assaults they had suffered. The fact that there has been no institutional discourse on such assaults within AKJP-Heidelberg until recently can have several reasons: Either the girls affected have not confided in anyone or exclusively in persons within their private environment. Or they have made corresponding disclosures in psychotherapeutic settings outside or within the "institute scene" of the AKJP-Heidelberg, but these disclosures were handled "confidentially" in such a way that there were no further consequences. At the level of the management and administration of the AKJP-Heidelberg, at any rate, one remained untroubled by such communications. In view of the hair-raising omissions with regard to known other case constellations, it cannot be assumed that there was any knowledge of how the abuses mentioned could have been classified in terms of professional ethics and criminal law. In the suspected case, psychotherapeutically dressed up "justifications" for these assaults on the basis of the interpretive power of the head of the institute would possibly have led to a similar paralysis of action as can be demonstrated in connection with the other case constellations. Doubts are also raised with regard to sufficient process/structural knowledge in the private and professional environment of the victims, since to our knowledge the indications of sexual boundary violations against adolescent patients* did not lead to sustained intervention action. Since it seems improbable that within the Heidelberg psychotherapy scene there was no knowledge of any incidents of sexual boundary violations by H. M. against adolescent patients for decades, the assumption suggests itself that a lack of process/structural knowledge was at least a relevant factor for possibly serious failures to act.

Sexual Relationships with Young Women During and After Psychotherapeutic Treatment

Due to the available data, we limit ourselves in this case constellation to an analysis of the knowledge base in the cases of R. R. and E. M. What is important here is first of all the question of which event knowledge was represented in which social systems. With regard to R. R., there were rumours according to which the patient was still a minor at the time of the conception of the common child with H. M. It is interesting in this case that within AKJP-Heidelberg and IPP-Heidelberg-Mannheim no attempt was made at any time to find out how old the patient was at the time of the pregnancy, whether she was still a patient of H. M. at the time of the pregnancy and whether the sexualization of the relationship had already begun before the end of the psychotherapy and/or when the patient was a minor. The still valid narrative of the contemporary witnesses consists in the fact that one knew about the child who repeatedly visited his father in work and that one alternatively assumed that the mother was a former patient or also a training candidate. A weakly developed knowledge of events, which was nourished not least by communications from H. M. and his secretary, haunted the rooms of the Institute, without initiatives being taken in the direction of a systematic clarification. We do not know whether actual event knowledge ever left the exclusive space of the abuse system constituted by H. M. It is not known, but strongly assumed on the basis of knowledge of other cases, that H. M. sexual the relationship with R. R. from the very beginning and harassed the adolescent with intimate questioning and touching from early stages of psychotherapy. It is important to note in this context that there appears to have been no serious effort from any side for a long time to ascertain, as best they could, regarding this highly suspicious but insufficiently substantiated event knowledge. There are, however, indications that the Youth Welfare Office became aware of the case, however, without a sustained critical discussion of the relationship between H. M. and R. R. having occurred. In the case of E. M. the question of event knowledge arises in a similar way. Due to the fact that in both cases children were born, there is at least certainty with regard to the indisputable event of sexual intercourse, which H. M. subsequently felt compelled to legitimize: The two women were adults and the sexual relationship did not begin until after the conclusion of the psychotherapy. In the case of E. M., H. M. apparently succeeded without major problems in denying the fact that there had been any psychotherapy at all and in spreading the fairy tale of the "diagnostic talks" without contradiction. The women victims, who naturally had knowledge of events, did not disclose this to the perpetrator, mainly for reasons of dependency. Both discourse knowledge and process/structural knowledge are clearly oriented towards the interpretation of event knowledge in these cases: Since it was apparently not possible to assert beyond doubt that E. M. had been in therapy with H. M. and that sexual contact had already occurred during therapy, it was necessary to switch to those reference discourses that dealt with the question of whether it was permissible to begin a sexual relationship with a patient *after the* end of psychotherapy. In this context, it seems particularly interesting that apparently no one had the idea of consulting the relevant institute files for reliable indications about the occasion, course and termination of E.M.'s psychotherapy with H. M. The information that E.M. had not been able to obtain from the institute's files was not reliable. The unverified information according to which H. M. made corresponding files disappear is rather not suitable to believe his version of events.

The obscuring of event knowledge, which was practiced not only by H. M. but also by the then chairwoman of the institute's board of directors, also contaminated the other bodies of knowledge: discourse knowledge seemed negotiable: Is it permissible to sleep with an ex-patient? Is a sexual relationship with an ex-patient legitimized after the fact if you marry her? Because the system of abuse defined by the sexual exploitation of the young woman, by the power of interpretation of the perpetrator, and by the pressure for secrecy (for example, the birth of the first child) was not recognized as such, no consensual discourse knowledge could be drawn upon in assessing the case. Of particular importance is the fact that both the Youth Welfare Office and the Criminal Investigation Department were investigating the case, so that, with recourse to appropriate process/structural knowledge, coordinated intervention action would have been likely. The helplessness of the authorities involved is conspicuous in view of the fact that an almost 60-year-old doctor and psychotherapist impregnates a young woman who has just become an adult, who had to cope with heavy biographical burdens and had been referred to him for psychotherapy. The question of whether this is legitimate was ultimately answered "yes" within the respective logics of the professional systems involved. The question of whether anything could be done about it resulted in a "no". Although H. M. had to give up his functions at the IPP-Heidelberg-Mannheim and resign as institute director of the AKJP-Heidelberg, he continued to work as a psychotherapist and expert witness, and the family system that emerged from the abusive relationship with his young patient remained largely untroubled by external challenges.

Despite manifold efforts, health insurance companies, professional associations and umbrella organizations remained unsuccessful in their attempt to withdraw the license to practice medicine from H. M. until 2013. It must be stated here that at least on the part of the IPP-Heidelberg-Mannheim and also in parts of the AKJP-Heidelberg, a degree of process/structural knowledge was available that at least opened up the theoretical possibility of imposing the necessary ban on H. M.'s profession. These initiatives ultimately failed due to an apparently insufficient knowledge of events, but possibly also due to a varying degree of willingness on the part of the addressed authorities to deal with the case. At least this can be concluded from the assessment of one of the experts we interviewed:

> *The professional associations are a thousand percent more committed to keeping their own stable clean, so to speak, I'll say; as opposed to many chambers.*

Within the AKJP-Heidelberg, the tactics of those who backed H. M. consisted in constantly referring to precisely this lack of knowledge of events: It was not legitimate to take action against H. M. if one acted on the basis of unproven allegations. It was part of this strategy to claim again and again that H. M.'s acts were not justiciable, that therefore criminal charges would be ineffective and that the victims were not willing to make any statements. In this way, there was a constant narrowing of the process knowledge to the decision about a criminal charge. A lack of process knowledge was expressed here, among other things, in the assumption that only the persons affected could file a criminal complaint themselves. In fact, however, every person is authorized to do so. From the introduction of the law in 1998, according to which sexual acts in the context of psychotherapies constitute a criminal offence, the relationship between H. M. and E. M. remained, at least from a legal point of view, natural. To our knowledge, there was no discourse about the fact that the event in question would have had to be assessed as a criminal offence retrospectively at least. Due to the increasing (professional) public discussion of sexual violence in general and sexual boundary violations in psychotherapy in particular, the conditions with regard to the availability of discourse knowledge and also process/structural knowledge changed, but this was not necessarily connected with improved intervention action – as the retrospective assessment of one of the experts we interviewed shows:

> *At the beginning of 98 there was actually nothing, it was a field that was uncultivated. Everyone was horrified when something came to light, but no one was able to act, not even us, because we somehow didn't know how to deal with it. And that's when ..., we all thought criminal law was the 'salvation', in inverted commas, and then found out that it wasn't like that at all.*

Knowledge developed and became established about the extent to which people are damaged by sexual violence, how perpetrator strategies function and what particular risks are associated with the psychotherapeutic setting. However, the body of knowledge in the case of H. M. remained fragmented, especially since the case was delegated further and further into a past that was rather regarded as historical. Requirements for action that had previously been considered urgent became less important, and knowledge of the event took on the form of a more or less relevant rumor. The fact that H. M.'s family regime and his psychotherapeutic practice continued to exist in parallel was seen as a problem only by a few people and at different times. It can be assumed that the rapidly developing public discourse on sexual violence made a considerable contribution to H. M.'s daughter deciding to file a complaint against her father, first with the medical association and subsequently with the criminal prosecution authorities. The criminal complaint of sexual abuse against his granddaughter paradigmatically combines event knowledge, discourse knowledge and process/structural knowledge on the part of H. M.'s daughter: Knowledge about the sexual abuse of the little girl, knowledge that it is a criminal offence, knowledge about help systems and the functioning of the justice system. The attempt initiated in this context to reactivate corresponding knowledge on the part of the ethics officer of the AKJP-Heidelberg failed, at least partially: From the court's point of view, the accusations made against H. M. remained minor from a legal point of view, time-barred or irrelevant for other reasons. Discourses, structures and procedures had changed over the decades, but H. M.'s acts committed in the context of the psychotherapeutic setting remained inaccessible to criminal sanction. However, the knowledge available within the AKJP Institute Heidelberg in the meantime about changed social discourses on sexual violence enabled – also on the basis of the "ZEIT" article – a sustainable reorganization and reinterpretation of the event knowledge. The astonishment expressed on all sides at H. M.'s acts is also the result of an increased social sensitivity with regard to sexual violence: downplaying, obfuscation and relativization are seen as completely inappropriate in view of the event and discourse knowledge now available. That it often takes decades to integrate bodies of knowledge is part of the destructive nature of sexual violence. To understand this, Rieske et al. (2018) concretization is important, according to which knowledge "does not [mean] incontrovertible facts or objectively understood truths. Event, discourse, process, and structural knowledge are social constructions because they are the result of interactive, institutional, and social processes" (p. 201). This understanding of knowledge also helps to explain barriers to action in dealing with the sexual relationships with teaching analysts and training candidates that have come to light.

Sexual Relationships with Teaching Analysts/Training Candidates

With regard to H. M.'s relationships with training candidates, there was a pronounced, albeit unsystematic, knowledge of events within the institute publics of AKJP-Heidelberg and IPP-Heidelberg-Mannheim from the beginning. The fact that he also had sexual relations with female students was also known, at least on the level of rumours. In connection with these constellations, it is above all the widespread lack of discourse knowledge that stands out. This affected fellow students as well as staff and those responsible for the institute, and also the women concerned themselves. The argument that there were no corresponding reference discourses at the time that would have made it possible to critically discuss such conditions falls short. There were snickers, there was indignation, there were moral sentiments, but there was no systematic reflection on how a psychotherapeutic institute dealt with the fact that its director apparently repeatedly had relationships with women who were doing their training at that institute. The concept of abstinence alone could have provided a starting point for appropriate discussions here. The finding of a collective refusal to appropriate potentially available discourse knowledge is therefore appropriate here.

This also applies to the women victims themselves, who were trained in a profession in which the ability to respect boundaries and strict adherence to abstinence rules are considered basic qualification criteria. This is also where the question of process/structural knowledge comes in: What is to be done when the setting of the teaching analysis is eroticized and these feelings are not only worked through symbolically but acted upon in real terms? At this point, the availability of reliable options for action is needed in order to prevent a development that carries the potential for lasting damage. Especially for the time before 1992/1993, it can be said that a low level of process/structure knowledge, both on the part of the affected women and on the part of their fellow students, can probably be linked to the lack of availability of reliable processes and structures.

One spoke with friends and colleagues and shared certain observations with one's teaching analyst, who remained meaningfully silent. If those responsible for the institute, both at AKJP-Heidelberg and at IPP-Heidelberg-Mannheim, consistently refuse over a long period of time to develop clear rules and procedures that prohibit intimate relationships between leadership/lecturers on the one hand and training candidates on the other, then a lack of process/structural knowledge on the part of all those involved is pre-programmed.

The fact that H. M. as the head of the institute naturally had little interest in establishing such regulations does not suffice as an argument for all other persons responsible for training who refrained from critically discussing such relationships and from working out appropriate regulations. What was true for sexual relationships with training candidates was even more true for erotic relationships with training analysands. Here, only the retreat to averted event knowledge helped: For example, with regard to B. U., for example, it seems hardly credible that the knowledge base in the two institutes IPP-Heidelberg-Mannheim and AKJP-Heidelberg was divided into two groups that could be clearly distinguished from each other: those who knew that B. U. was in training analysis with H. M., but did not know that the two were involved with each other. And those who knew that the two were involved with each other but did not know that she was in training analysis with him.

The suspicion suggests itself that the lack of availability of process/structure knowledge leads to a fearful defence against event knowledge: If I don't know how to act, I prefer to ignore cues to possible action requirements. Of course, there was discourse knowledge that a sexual relationship between a teaching analyst and a teaching analysand is a serious offence, but the lack of process knowledge (i.e. knowledge of what I should do if I have knowledge of such a relationship) no longer weighs so heavily if I deny the existence of this relationship or retreat to the secrecy of the psychoanalytic setting. The picture that presents itself, then, is one of fragmented, contaminated, or wholly immature bodies of knowledge that permanently limited the ability to act of all those involved in the institute. In this context, reference should be made above all to the failure of the staff, lecturers and teaching analysts in both institutes to assume responsibility.

We do not know what prompted about four to five affected women towards the end of 1992 to confide in a supervisor of the IPP-Heidelberg-Mannheim and to report sexual exploitation by H. M. in the context of teaching analyses and training relationships. We do not know how long they had been aware of the damaging and destructive nature of their relationships with H. M. at this point; but it seems clear that they had all come to the realization that H. M.'s behavior was not remotely compatible with an appropriate professional ethos and that this warranted a complaint to the board of IPP-Heidelberg-Mannheim. The fact that they took this route is evidence of the existence of appropriate process/structural knowledge.

This shows how discourse, process/structure and event knowledge combine to form effective action. The victims refrain from pressing charges and attach great importance to strictly maintaining their anonymity. With recourse to their respective bodies of knowledge, they go their own way of coping, which is different from the way the two institutes AKJP-Heidelberg and IPP-Heidelberg-Mannheim are faced with as soon as they become aware of the reports of the affected women.

Similar to the cases of R. R. and E. M., the permanent lack of event knowledge also opens up problematic room for interpretation, which was not least filled by H. M.'s allegations: In a total of three cases, he had only entered into sexual relations with teaching analysands after the completion of the teaching analyses. The institutional handling of sexual boundary violations is almost bound to fail if all initiatives are traced back to the narrative of the perpetrator: Is it legitimate to engage in sexual relations with a teaching analyst after the completion of a teaching analysis? Who actually initiated these relationships? Are they not simply relationships between adults?

The knowledge available in the two institutes is subsequently comparable to that concerning the case of E. M. in particular. Under the assumption that the relationships are serious abstinence violations, corresponding notifications are made to health insurance companies, medical associations, professional associations and umbrella organizations. However, because there is a lack of sufficient knowledge of the events, H. M. can threaten with libel suits, so that the hands of the various instances remain tied. Factions, by which H. M. is protected, can retreat without major hardships to the question whether something illegal had happened at all.

The further development proceeds as described above in the case of the young female patients who had been impregnated by H. M.: Increasing social discourse knowledge; establishment of structures that form anchor points for process/structure knowledge and reorganization of event knowledge in the course of the court case against H. M. and on the basis of the "ZEIT" article.

In all of the case constellations described here, it becomes apparent that a professional approach to (suspected cases of) sexual violence in the context of psychotherapeutic settings and institutions consists of agreeing on ethical standards (discourse knowledge), developing and making transparent procedures in the case of assumptions and suspicions (process/structural knowledge), and seeking ways to obtain the most well-founded knowledge possible about the events in question (event knowledge). Such knowledge not only provides a suitable frame of reference for intervention action, but also has a preventive effect in many ways.

8.4 Traumatized Institutions

The concept of "traumatized institutions", whose empirical-scientific foundation is still pending, is suitable as a further background frame for the events surrounding H. M.'s boundary violations at the AKJP-Heidelberg and at the IPP-Heidelberg-Mannheim, but which was developed on the basis of extensive experience in the counselling of institutions (Enders, 2004). As a result of the (partial) disclosure of sexual violence "within their own ranks", institutions often show a pattern of reaction that is phenomenologically reminiscent of the symptomatology of traumatized people. Enders (2004) described conclusive analogies between individual stress reactions and institutional events as a result of the "shock experience" of a disclosure of sexual violence within one's own area of responsibility. Institutions in which sexual assaults have been committed by the management are particularly at risk for such massive reactions.

In the examination of the events at the AKJP Institute in Heidelberg in particular, clear features of such an institutional shock reaction can be demonstrated (cf.

also Burka et al., 2019). The reference to analogies to individual post-traumatic stress reactions also makes clear which intervention requirements existed in different phases of the institution's development and which failures can be demonstrated in this regard.

The analysis undertaken here is initially limited to purely phenomenological evidence of the presence of the post-traumatic symptom triad at the AKJP Institute Heidelberg, so that we focus primarily on intrusive phenomena, symptoms of overexcitement and avoidance behaviour (cf. Fischer & Riedesser, 2009).

Intrusion: Intrusive symptoms, which manifest themselves, among other things, as so-called "flashbacks", are associated with an involuntary, emotionally very stressful recollection of the traumatic event. To put it briefly, the individual is "caught up" again and again by these unprocessed experiences. The risk of such stressful episodes is increased by associated trigger stimuli. With regard to the institutes AKJP-Heidelberg and IPP-Heidelberg-Mannheim, a transfer of these psychological events to institutional dynamics seems immediately evident: While until 1992/1993 all indications of "pathological" stress could be kept "under cover", so to speak, by various defence strategies (and the institutions themselves remained largely unaffected by associated stress reactions), the "clinical picture" of the institutions changed massively as a result of the crisis of disclosure. (The loss of superficial functionality through the disclosure crisis is a phenomenon frequently observed in abuse victims.) At first, it appears as if the strains on the system were less due to the boundary transgressions of the head of the institution than to their exposure. In the further course, the picture of institutions that do not come to rest presents itself. The "unprocessed trauma" – activated by various triggers – repeatedly breaks into the institutional consciousness and necessitates coping action in this regard. It is interesting here that the IPP-Heidelberg-Mannheim – in a figurative sense – repeatedly acts as a "trigger" for the AKJP-Heidelberg by putting its finger in the wound of the unresolved issue. Expert opinions signed by H. M., complaints from parents or reminders from former training candidates cause intrusive reactions within AKJP-Heidelberg, which make it necessary to activate "practiced" defense mechanisms. Intrusive symptoms are – if the stressful event is not sufficiently processed – independent of the passage of time.[1] What applies to individuals can be seen in the reaction of AKJP-Heidelberg to the court case against H. M. and to the publication of the "ZEIT" article. One could speak here of classic triggers that suddenly make the pain of institutional burden immediately perceptible again. Unprepared, the system is caught up with events believed to be long past.

[1] "Once an ethical boundary is destroyed, the effects reverberate. Recovery of trust in oneself and others occurs gradually, if at all" (Burka et al., 2019, p. 261).

The intrusive character becomes apparent in the fact that it is not just a matter of mere recollection, but of hard-to-control affects that accompany these memories that are perceived as imposed.

The affective dimension is accentuated even more strongly in the second main symptom of post-traumatic stress disorder, the so-called "hyperarousal". This refers to a habitualized over-excitement or overexcitability as a result of the traumatic experience. The "smallest" stress stimuli cause strong emotional reactions; the affected person is "constantly on guard" because he or she fears that something bad might happen. The underlying experience of this symptom manifestation is the loss of belief in an environment that is experienced as safe. The metaphorical content of this psychological constellation in relation to the AKJP-Heidelberg is evident: Through the (partial) exposure of the transgressions of the head of the institute, a feeling of comprehensive existential danger breaks into the system. What could previously be dismissed with humour, trivialization or non-perception suddenly condenses into an event that affects everyone: the existence of the system is called into question (just as traumatic experiences can call into question the life and survival of the victims).

The secure job is just as endangered as the predictable training path, professional identities are attacked, the framework of the training institute experienced as reliable suddenly becomes fragile and incalculable (cf. Burka et al., 2019; Sandler & Godley, 2004). At this point, certain protagonists of AKJP-Heidelberg represent a faction that subordinates everything to the primacy of institutional survival. Clinically formulated, one could speak here of a peritraumatic emergency reaction.

In fact, the institute survives. However, the transformation of the survival reaction into a reflexive consideration of the trauma event does not succeed – from an institutional point of view. A clear expression of this lack of transformation is the institutional hyperarousal: violent affective reactions can be reactivated at any time because the feeling of a fundamental existential threat to the system continues to nest in its foundations. This is shown by an account of a colleague at the conference on the occasion of the 50th anniversary of the AKJP Institute in Heidelberg: "I can't remember the content, but it became very, very dense, very emotional. She then told how bad it was from her point of view. She burst into tears, that was quite intense. And she couldn't talk any more for a while. Yes … It was such an event … That's how it always happened. And then we talk about it for a while and then we don't."

A few years later, when the AKJP Institute in Heidelberg was commissioned to carry out a scientific investigation into the "Causa H. M.", a psychotherapist reported the following observations:

So I was thinking at this general meeting, and I'm not so prone to trauma, and they're all traumatized and stuff, I'm very cautious about that. But that's when I thought, sometimes I think there goes – so nobody rests until they're all damaged.

"One" feels attacked at every opportunity and "one" cannot open oneself to reflexive discourse, because with every discussion of the "Causa H. M." the feeling of existential threat is associated (cf. Burka et al., 2019). The AKJP-Heidelberg survives, but it can never be completely certain of its existence, because unprocessed things point to the fact that not only human life, but also the functionality of institutions could be permanently threatened. The extent and variety of emotional reactions occurring in the aftermath of the court case against H. M. and the publication of the "ZEIT" article, in the context of members' meetings and in the course of our interviews, point to the potential of "over-excitement" represented within the system. The discourse figure, according to which the existence of the institute would be endangered by a scientific processing of the "Causa H. M.", transforms the fundamental existential fear onto a discursive level, but at the same time neglects an important aspect of overcoming trauma: The pain of processing does not originate in the processing itself, but in what has to be processed.

The third aspect of the symptom triad of post-traumatic stress disorder can also be clearly demonstrated at the level of the institutional system AKJP-Heidelberg: Avoidance. In the mental household of people affected by trauma, avoidance plays a significant role in the context of coping (Mosser & Schlingmann, 2013). This strategy becomes pathological when it significantly restricts everyday life: No longer going to certain places, withdrawing from social contacts, avoiding conversations about certain topics. Avoidance is not pathological per se, but in therapeutic treatment it must be considered from the point of view of its (dys-)functional character. Without doubt, avoidance is an important element in the repertoire of institutional defense mechanisms that AKJP-Heidelberg has appropriated in connection with the boundary transgressions of its institute director. However, the refusal of any systematic intervention to protect victims over a period of 18 years should not be understood in terms of post-traumatic avoidance. After the disclosure crisis, the institutional picture is one of a competing dynamic between activity and avoidance. Put simply, one could say that – in analogy to individual trauma coping – the strategy of avoidance can always establish itself up to that point where a "trigger" triggers an intrusive event that leads to the imposed breakdown of avoidance. Avoidance serves functionality by enabling attention to the "real" tasks of the system. Retrospectively, it can be said with regard to the AKJP-Heidelberg that (almost) every effort towards confrontation was at the same time connected with weighty ambitions towards avoidance. Symptomatic here appears the course of the group "Past – Present – Future", which apparently lost itself in a mode of rationalization, at the end of which there was no longer any talk of H. M. at all. In the analysis of the systemic events, the difficulty arises to judge to what extent the avoidance of confrontation serves the functionality of the system. This question is highly topical in view of the commissioning of the scientific inquiry and therefore requires intensive reflection.

In their trauma processing, individuals navigate between coping with life and painful confrontation, whereby the success of this process depends on finding a balance in this respect, which proves to be accessible to reflexive observation. Exemplarily, one could ask on the level of the system: Does avoidance rather serve the maintenance of functionality or the defense against (personal) guilt? In view of the fact that there were persons who knowingly tolerated the abuse systems initiated by H. M., this question is by no means insignificant.

In addition, there is the attempt to avoid disclosure, since this is what makes everything really serious. In that an institution is – metaphorically speaking – "traumatized" by the exposure of sexual violence, the system dynamics described here lead to limitations in the institutional ability to perceive, to difficulties in understanding contexts, to a corresponding fragmentation of institutional memory representation, and to an overall damaged ability of the institution to act (Burka et al., 2019; Weick et al., 2016). Enders (2004) speaks of "institutional dissociation" in this context. These phenomena can be demonstrated without difficulty in the context of the AKJP-Heidelberg's handling of the "Causa H. M.". Therefore, in retrospect – despite all the limitations regarding the transfer of individual stress reactions to institutional systems – the application of the diagnosis of a "traumatized institution" at the AKJP-Heidelberg suggests itself.

Analogous to clinical phenomena that can be detected in individuals, institutional stress reactions are by no means to be understood context-free. Therefore, the metaphor of the "traumatized institution" offers less of an explanation for the processes at the AKJP Institute Heidelberg, but rather a hermeneutic framework into which observed phenomena can be (retrospectively) classified.

Background and Functioning of Structural Prevention

9

Before formulating some recommendations for a structural prevention in the AKJP-Institute Heidelberg, some basic remarks are necessary to justify the necessity of preventive considerations and to convey some basic orientations in this respect:

- The case of H. M. opens up the possibility of generating important insights into certain risks associated with psychotherapeutic work. Regardless of the question of whether H. M. is an extreme case, the abundance and heterogeneity of the verifiable acts alone point to a variety of potential dangers that must be taken seriously and addressed in the context of preventive considerations: Sexual boundary violations towards children and adolescents in the context of psychotherapies and assessments; sexualization of psychotherapeutic settings with adult patients, partly with the aim of preparing physical sexual interactions and establishing sexual relationships; sexualization of training settings (here specifically: teaching analysis, supervision), partly with the aim of preparing physical sexual interactions and establishing sexual relationships. Another constellation that could not be directly proven in the context of H. M., but which occurs frequently according to an expert we interviewed, is the sexualization of contacts with parents of therapy children (see also Schleu et al., 2018). It is known both from the literature and from indications in our interviews that the scenarios listed here are by no means to be reduced to the person of H. M., but are also produced by other psychotherapists with a frequency that is not to be neglected.
- The report presented here is suitable as a frame of reference to which discourses on (sexual) boundary violations can be referred both within and outside

P. Caspari et al., *At some point there has to be peace and quiet!*,
https://doi.org/10.1007/978-3-658-39785-2_9

AKJP-Heidelberg. It can therefore itself be used as an instrument for preventive efforts.

- If we look at current discourses on institutional prevention of (sexual) violence, two different guiding concepts seem to be used, depending on the professional or organizational orientation: While prevention in the pedagogical field is unmistakably under the primacy of protection and therefore the instrument of the protection concept has established itself as the main strategy for corresponding initiatives (cf. Caspari, 2021b; Kappler et al., 2019; Oppermann et al., 2018), in the medical and psychotherapeutic field one refers primarily to the dimension of ethics (cf. Schleu, 2021), which has led to the codification of ethical guidelines and the establishment of ethics committees. In terms of discourse history, parallel developments seem to emerge here with a strikingly low degree of reciprocal references. One reason for this may be that the pedagogical field is primarily (but not only) related to children and adolescents, while ethical discussions in the psychotherapeutic field mainly refer to (sexual) boundary violations against adult patients. As a currently observable preliminary "collateral damage" of the disconnectedness of these two lines of discourse, structural and content-related deficits regarding the prevention of sexual exploitation of children and adolescents in the psychotherapeutic-medical field can be identified (Kappler et al., 2019; Kaufman & Erooga, 2016).
- Investing time, energy and money in the prevention of incidents that are considered to be rather rare generates ambivalences and contradictions. One of the most important findings of the present research is that failures in detection and processing in connection with the "Causa H. M." were largely due to institutional and personal "functional pragmatism". To put it pointedly: One had better, respectively more important things to do. It could be shown that this functional orientation was easily compatible with the fact that an institute director could sexually exploit people in the context of the psychotherapy institute over a long period of time. Structural prevention can presumably only succeed if it is not seen as a rarely occurring but emotionally highly charged "orchid problem", but if a sustainable integration of topics such as "sexuality", "body", "shaping of closeness and distance", "abstinence", "shame", "power and dependency", "psychological violence", "sexual violence", etc. into the general quality development discourse of a psychotherapy institute is achieved.
- This also implies a view according to which it is not a matter of preventing individuals from living out their sexual perversions, but of recognising constellations of power and dependency that are in principle susceptible to narcissistic self-appreciation and abuse of any kind.

The recommendations formulated below represent an attempt to integrate the above-mentioned largely separate prevention discourses from the educational field on the one hand and from the medical-psychotherapeutic field on the other. We choose this approach not only because an institute for child and adolescent psychotherapy understandably has important overlaps with pedagogical institutions, since the fundamental objective in both, is to support the development of young people. Moreover, it should not be overlooked that a prevention discourse has been developing in Germany for more than ten years, which, although originally primarily aimed at preventing sexual violence in pedagogical settings, has since undergone a variety of differentiations that can in principle be used by all institutions and organizations in which people are cared for, taught and treated (Kappler et al., 2019).

Integration means: making connections between concepts such as "abstinence" and "ethics" on the one hand and "protection" or "concepts of protection" on the other. In our interviews we also encountered, in part, a certain scepticism towards an "over-regulation" of psychoanalysis. The assumption that rules and concepts could be used to organize human behavior in the context of psychotherapy in such a way as to significantly reduce the likelihood of boundary violations was qualified as too optimistic. Such reservations are important because they can be identified as part of a certain professional culture which – to put it simply – is less interested in regulations on the outside than in inner processes, relational representations, projections, transferences and countertransferences. The sometimes reported assessment that training analyses and supervision are the "structural qualification instruments" that can make the most significant contribution to preventing damaging psychotherapy processes also fits in with this fundamental attitude. Far from casting doubt on this perspective in principle, it is nevertheless worth pointing out that H. M.'s assaults were obviously alluded to or clearly named in supervisions, training analyses and psychotherapies over years and decades, without this discourse system, which primarily refers to itself and withdraws to the primacy of confidentiality, having contributed in any significant way to ending sexual exploitation.[1] The question therefore arises: How can the developmental processes that take place in the context of teaching analyses and supervision be integrated, if necessary, into structures that enable reliable and effective intervention action?

[1] Interesting here, for example, is a critical remark by Wruck from 1998 on the question of "how one can methodically help the analyst to recognize and discuss the danger instead of acting it out, that is, to avoid abuse. As far as I am informed, the main idea at present for solving the problem is to run the teaching analysis sufficiently deep. In view of 1000 h and more, however, this seems to reach its limits". (Wruck, 1998, p. 340)

Organizational prevention must also take into account the fact that structures and instruments have long existed in psychotherapy umbrella organizations as well as in the psychotherapists' and doctors' associations that are in principle suitable for addressing sexual boundary violations in the context of psychotherapy. There are ethics and arbitration committees in different structural contexts, which use different procedures in the event of complaints. In addition, with the nationally active Ethics Association, there is a body that acts as an important point of reference both at the level of intervention and at the level of prevention, qualification and scientific contextualization of the problem, both for concrete incidents and for a general improvement in the security of action in this regard. Since sexual interactions in the context of psychotherapies have constituted a criminal offence in the StGB since 1998, this also opens up the possibility of criminal charges and thus the involvement of investigative authorities.

Despite the instances and instruments briefly listed here, there is still a need for development. These have to do above all with certain characteristics of sexual violence, which not only have to do with pronounced feelings of shame and fear on the part of the victims, but also with considerable difficulties in interpreting situations, interactions and relationship constellations correctly and deriving the appropriate consequences from hints, reports and observations. These serious problems can be proven in the analysis of the case of H. M. in great frequency and manifold variations and they will also appear in some form in every (suspicious) case in the future. For this reason, too, there is a need to integrate a more "relationship-oriented prevention" (in the context of seminars, teaching analyses and supervision) into a structural prevention, which should serve as its functional frame of reference.

Preventive efforts presuppose an awareness of the fact that within the framework of a training institute for child and adolescent psychotherapy there are different risk scenarios which require different approaches, especially in the context of intervention:

- (Sexual) violence against children and adolescents by trainees or colleagues in the context of psychotherapy. The case of H. M. indicates a part of the possible spectrum of boundary violations in this regard. This also includes, for example, shaming through invasive or embarrassing questions.
- Sexualization of the relationship to parents of therapy children. H. M.'s assessment in the context of a supervision, according to which a mother appeared to him to be "sexually needy", could have triggered many questions and reflections, e.g.: How does a psychotherapist determine the assessment that parents are "sexually needy" and what special requirements result from this for their own contact with these parents?

- Sexualization of therapeutic relationships with adult patients. The "classical" discourse of abstinence in psychoanalysis is directed at this constellation. Due to the variety of possible and conceivable scenarios, important differentiations are needed here (e.g., on the question of when the "latency period" ends after the end of psychotherapy). It seems important to us to be aware that the psychoanalytic setting has a serious potential for damaging intimacy, transgressions and abuse of power. The fact that this was called into doubt by several interview partners, we interpret as a symptom for the necessity of preventive discourses.
- Sexualization of relationships with supervisees and teaching analysands. Even if these groups of people are not to be qualified as "sick" in the clinical sense and the sexualization of the therapeutic relationship would therefore not prevent their "healing", a clear ethical positioning arises from the problematic asymmetry of power between the participants. Supervisees and teaching analysands open themselves to their "abstinent" psychotherapists and are in a relationship of dependence to them due to the demands of their training. The launching of psychological, physical and/or sexual boundary violations therefore constitutes an abuse of power. The persistence of such a situation and the corresponding damaging effects on the lives of the victims can be paradigmatically traced using the case of H. M.

In view of the variety of possible potential dangers, we consider one more hint to be of particular importance, which we derive from a remark in one of our interviews. One colleague pointed out to us that her/his colleagues would never report feelings of infatuation towards patients in the context of supervision, because in this case they would have to fear that their suitability for the psychotherapeutic profession would be fundamentally called into question. This comment surprised us, especially as it should be seen in the context of some similar comments from other interviews. It refers to the difference between the symbolic level of certain manifestations of feelings on the one hand, which usually emerges in the context of countertransference, and the acting out of such feelings on the other. On the basis of this differentiation, feelings of infatuation on the part of the psychotherapist represent therapeutic "material", the reflection of which within the framework of supervision contributes in a constitutive way to the development of the therapeutic process and to the success of the therapy. It is therefore not the feelings of infatuation that represent a problem related to the profession, but the failure to bring them up in the supervisory setting. It is immediately evident that serious requirements for prevention arise from this observation. These would have to relate, among other things, to the question of how it can be possible to design supervision in such a way that supervisees feel able to reflect on such fundamental material without fear.

Not least because of this last observation, we see prevention needs in institutes for child and adolescent psychotherapy primarily in three areas that can be roughly differentiated from one another, namely (1) internal procedures and structures, (2) qualification and (3) external cooperation.

10 Recommendations

10.1 Internal Procedures and Structures

Risk and Potential Analysis

There is a need for a fundamental understanding within the institution about possible risk potentials for (sexual) transgressions and abuse of power in the context of one's own institution. This should not be confused with a paranoid search for all conceivable horror scenarios, but should result in an openly communicable agreement on everything that preventive efforts should be directed at. Fundamental here is the differentiation into various dangerous situations described above. In addition, there is a need for an open discourse about situations in which one felt insecure as a staff member, training candidate or manager with regard to the observance of boundaries or the possibly illegitimate exercise of power. The risk analysis must be coupled with an analysis of potential: this refers to the identification of structures, competences and knowledge that have already been anchored in the institution in the sense of successful prevention. Here one can also refer to experiences in which the usefulness of one's own preventive efforts has already been proven.

Mission Statement

Not least because of the experience gained from the risk analysis, the institutional awareness of possible hazards and the resulting responsibility for all professional groups working in the institution should find expression in the Institute's mission statement. The report presented here can be used as a starting point for making visible one's own reflexivity with regard to this topic.

P. Caspari et al., *At some point there has to be peace and quiet!*,
https://doi.org/10.1007/978-3-658-39785-2_10

The mission statement also serves as an expression of a certain organizational ethic, which should be an ongoing task of the Institute's members.

Confidential Counsellors

In the context of preventive considerations, it may also be possible to redefine the function of internal confidential counsellors. What is important here is first of all an institutional commitment to the necessity and importance of such a position, which results in the appropriate provision of resources and fundamental support from the management and board level. Above all, the role of the confidential counsellors as contact persons for both the intervention and the prevention of (sexual) violence and abuse of power in the area of responsibility of the institute must be clearly defined (see the ethics guidelines of the AKJP-Heidelberg).[1] Contact details and functions of the confidential counsellors must be actively and possibly recurrently publicized within the institute in order to increase the likelihood of their being called upon. In all likelihood, this will be accompanied by a high degree of willingness on the part of all institute staff and members to perceive problematic situations as such and to engage in a responsible discourse.

10.2 Qualification

Acquisition of Discourse and Structural/Process Knowledge Our analysis has shown that both serious deficits in the evaluation of indications and clues as well as pronounced uncertainties with regard to necessary interventions led to the enabling of H. M.'s acts and prevented their detection over long periods of time. Immediate qualification requirements are derived from this, which refer to the acquisition or expansion of discourse knowledge as well as process/structural knowledge. Behind these general terms, complex questions are hidden, which, among other things, deal with the following: "How do we define boundary violations, abstinence violations, abuse of power and sexual violence?" And, "What can I do if I have the impression that colleagues are committing sexual boundary violations or exploiting their power at the expense of patients or colleagues? Which authorities can/must I use as contact persons in such cases and what are their tasks?" Discourse knowledge is closely linked to discussions about one's own professional ethics.

[1] http://www.andreas-renzel.de/mediapool/131/1313656/data/Ethikleitinien_24-11-19.pdf.

These should be conducted within the framework of obligatory ethics seminars and in supervision, but also in teaching analyses. This is not only a question of the extent to which one is at risk as a candidate of committing boundary violations that are incompatible with the professional ethos of psychotherapists. Rather, an open discourse must also be established about the working methods of colleagues (especially with regard to their proximity-distance behaviour and their handling of power) and the working methods of supervisors, lecturers and teaching analysts. The fact that such an open discourse is not experienced as denunciation is an atmospheric requirement that must be met with the help of strategies based on organizational ethics. The imparting of discourse knowledge also includes information about criminal law framework conditions as well as aspects of child welfare endangerment. At the same time, this also opens up access to the area of process/structural knowledge. This relates above all to the possibilities of intervention.

It is important to note that (prospective) psychotherapists cannot be expected to know all institutional and official procedural channels in the event of a possible suspicion of an abstinence violation or sexual abuse. As a rule, process/structural knowledge can be limited to knowing the internally prescribed reporting channels and being able to use them reliably. However, a broader process/structure knowledge is to be expected on the part of the confidential counsellors and the management staff, since their intervention action must in many cases point beyond the boundaries of their own institution. The case of H. M. is also a reminder of the need to establish procedures which must take effect in the event of suspicion against the institution's management.

Within the framework of prevention, binding contexts should be established within which the qualification requirements described here are implemented.

Declaration of Commitment and Code of Conduct A further aspect of qualification (which at the same time can also be attributed to the internal procedures described above) could refer to the instruments of the declaration of commitment and the code of conduct, which are now common in the pedagogical context. The ethics guidelines of the AKJP-Heidelberg already offer sensible stipulations in this regard, although there are still questions about the creation of binding force (e.g. by signing) and the concretization of behavioural norms.

Even if it can be assumed that psychotherapists are reluctant to commit themselves to certain explicitly formulated rules of conduct, it should nevertheless be considered whether self-commitment declarations and codes of conduct could serve as an orientation framework for both professional and organizational ethical specifications. Possible profits of such instruments could be that they function as a starting point for discursive assurances, e.g. in the context of ethics seminars, and furthermore expand the spectrum of possible interventions in cases of suspicion. (Possible example: If it is stipulated that the door of the therapy room may not be locked from the inside when one is inside with a patient, then corresponding violations can be problematized without having to raise the accusation of a sexual boundary violation at the same time).

Another aspect to be anchored here relates to the reflection of power and dependency aspects within training structures. The potential for abuse of power must be explicitly addressed in the code of conduct and the declaration of commitment.

10.3 External Cooperation

Complaints Procedure

Complaints procedures are an important instrument, which in part also belong to the area of internal procedures and structures. However, they require an indispensable structural supplement that opens up a path to the outside of the institute. It could be shown within the framework of this investigation that the AKJP Institute Heidelberg was for a long time almost exclusively dependent on impulses from outside in order to critically discuss, uncover and come to terms with H. M.'s deeds. This makes it clear that there is a need for the implementation of structural elements that point beyond the boundaries of the institute, but also beyond the boundaries of the "psychotherapy scene", both in prevention and in intervention.

The establishment of complaints procedures should make it easier for both patients and their parents to complain both within the institute (as a rule to the confidential counsellors or the management) and outside the institute in the event of experienced transgressions or perceived abuse of power. For this purpose, it is important that patients and their parents are informed actively and in an understandable way about the possibilities of complaint (at the ethics association or at the professional associations). In addition, the installation of an ombudsperson should be considered, who fulfils the function of an external complaints office. Complaint possibilities must also exist for training candidates, so that they can react to violations of boundaries and abuse of power, especially in the context of teaching analyses and supervision. This also requires reliable contact persons both within and outside the institute. A functioning complaints management not only includes active information about the possibilities of complaints, but also the communication of an institutional attitude, according to which complaints are in principle desired, in order to further develop quality assurance and organizational ethics.

In thinking about this, a discourse is needed about the fact that the psychotherapeutic relationship, by its very nature, has a certain inherent potential for offenses and disappointments, so that occasions for a variety of complaints can be derived from it. The fact that such a discourse will not bring easy and quick solutions cannot be an alibi for not conducting it. At least – and not only – the case of H. M. points out that the exclusive, clandestine setting of psychoanalysis gives the psychotherapist a high degree of interpretative power, which can lead to its abuse. Therefore, there is a need for a structural opening of this setting to the outside, which is compatible with the interactional and emotional demands of psychotherapy.

Procedural Guidelines

At the heart of all prevention are established procedural guidelines for the "case of emergency". As already indicated above, knowledge of the existence of such procedural guidelines increases the willingness of all actors in an institution not to ignore possible anomalies, indications or "gut feelings" simply because they do not know what to do with them. Analogous to the complaints procedure, procedural guidelines consist of internally and externally oriented elements. A rough distinction can be made to the effect that most employees and training candidates initially tend to make use of internal instances when they make conspicuous observations or receive corresponding information. It is also important here that internal responsibilities are named within the framework of the procedural guidelines, among other things with the aim of avoiding free-floating rumours and insufficiently reflected actionism.

As described above, the internal responsibility for dealing with possible boundary violations or suspected abuse of power will lie with the confidential counsellors and the management. Their task is subsequently to cooperate with external bodies both in the assessment of the information that has become known and in the possibly necessary implementation of further intervention steps. At the level of case assessment, these can be the ethics committees of psychotherapeutic professional or umbrella associations, or specialist counselling centres against sexual violence, which represent a "structural outside" of the "psychotherapy scene". If further intervention is deemed necessary on the basis of an externally validated case assessment, the spectrum of external cooperation partners can be expanded to include, for example, youth welfare offices or law enforcement agencies. In any case, the inclusion of an external perspective is indispensable for a well-founded handling of assumptions or suspicions regarding (sexual) transgressions and/or abuse of power.

Networks

It seems important that the Institute is not only organized within psychotherapeutic associations, but that reliable networks are also established with institutions that are not genuinely psychotherapeutically oriented, but which can open up helpful perspectives for the present context. Such institutions could be, for example, specialist counselling centres against sexual violence, sexual education institutions or youth welfare offices, which normally also network with judicial authorities or the police, for example, within the framework of regional working groups, in order to develop coordinated procedures for dealing with (suspected) cases of sexual violence.

The great advantage of these networks is the establishment of personal contacts, which can be used both for the further development of prevention and for increased certainty of action in the case of intervention. Especially as an Institute for Child and Adolescent Psychotherapy, valuable synergies can be expected through cooperation with institutions outside the psychotherapeutic and medical fields, which can contribute to the consolidation of a preventive culture in the Institute. For example, the commissioning of non-psychotherapeutic lecturers within the framework of the qualification of training candidates and employees can be considered, as well as the referral of children, adolescents and parents to offers that could meaningfully complement the work carried out at the Institute.

The extent to which the recommendations proposed here lead to a prevention concept or to an extension of the institute's own ethical guidelines is a question that should be clarified in the AKJP-Heidelberg against the background of the most promising possible communicability of preventive requirements.

It is important that the considerations developed in this context are reliably and generally known in order to have a frame of reference for an organizational ethics related to the AKJP-Heidelberg. According to Wenger (2008), such codifications are to be understood in the sense of an element of a sequence of *reification* and *participation,* i.e.: each agreement fixed in writing is both the result of a participatory discourse and the starting point for the classification of future experiences and for the identification of needs for change, which in turn lead to new codifications. Prevention is thus a constantly evolving dialectical process that depends on binding structures. The present report may be understood as a useful impulse for such a process.

References

Aisslinger, M., & Lebert, S. (2018, August 16). Das kranke System des Doktor F. Wie ein renommierter Heidelberger Therapeut seine Patientinnen missbrauchte und jahrzehntelang von Kollegen gedeckt wurde. *Die Zeit*, 34. https://www.zeit.de/2018/34/missbrauch-psychotherapie-patientinnen-schuld-system. Accessed: 27. Feb. 2021.

AKJP. (n.d.). https://akjp-hd.de/

Araji, S. K. (1997). *Sexually aggressive children. Coming to understand them.*

Bange, D., & Deegener, G. (1996). *Sexueller Mißbrauch an Kindern. Ausmaß, Hintergründe, Folgen*. Beltz Psychologie-Verl.-Union.

Bauriedl, T. (1998). Ohne Abstinenz stirbt die Psychoanalyse. Über die Unvereinbarkeit von Psychoanalyse und Körpertherapie. *Forum der Psychoanalyse, 14*, 342–363.

Becker-Fischer, M., & Fischer, G. (1995). Sexuelle Übergriffe in Psychotherapie und Psychiatrie. Forschungsbericht des Instituts für Psychotraumatologie Freiburg. In *Bundesministerium für Familie, Senioren, Frauen und Jugend. Materialien zur Frauenpolitik* (Bd. 51).

Becker-Fischer, M., & Fischer, G. (1996). *Sexueller Mißbrauch in der Psychotherapie – Was tun? Orientierungshilfen für Therapeuten und interessierte Patienten (Thema)*. Asanger.

Becker-Fischer, M., & Fischer, G. (2018). *Sexuelle Übergriffe in Psychotherapie und Psychiatrie. Orientierungshilfen für Therapeut und Klientin* (5. Aufl.). Asanger.

Bion, W. R. (1991). *Learning from experience* (Maresfield library, 3. print). Karnac.

Bion, W. R. (2013). *Lernen durch Erfahrung*. Suhrkamp.

Bittner, G. (1998). Liebe in der Analyse – Ein Fall für den Staatsanwalt? Überlegungen zum „Gesetzesvorhaben gegen sexuellen Missbrauch in der Psychotherapie". *Forum der Psychoanalyse,14*, 301–311.

Blumer, H. (1973). Der methodologische Standort des symbolischen Interaktionismus. In Arbeitsgruppe Bielefelder Soziologen (Hrsg.), *Alltagswissen, Interaktion und gesellschaftliche Wirklichkeit* (S. 80–101). Rowohlt. http://hehl-rhoen.de/pdf/Philosopie/blumer%20-%20interaktionismus.pdf. Accessed: 19. Febr. 2021.

P. Caspari et al., *At some point there has to be peace and quiet!*,
https://doi.org/10.1007/978-3-658-39785-2

Bohnsack, R. (2000). Dokumentarische Methode und sozialwissenschaftliche Hermeneutik. *Zeitschrift für Erziehungswissenschaft, 6*, 550–570.

Bossi, J. (1994). Empirische Untersuchungen, Psychodynamik und Folgeschäden. In K. M. Bachmann & W. Bröker (Hrsg.), *Sexueller Mißbrauch in Psychotherapie und Psychiatrie* (S. 45–72). Huber.

Bronfenbrenner, U., Lüscher, K., & Cranach, A. v. (Hrsg.). (1981). *Die Ökologie der menschlichen Entwicklung. Natürliche und geplante Experimente* (Sozialwissenschaften, 1. Aufl.). Klett-Cotta.

Burka, J. B. (2008). Psychic fallout from breach of confidentiality. *Contemporary Psychoanalysis, 44*(2), 177–198.

Burka, J., Sowa, A., Baer, B. A., Brandes, C. E., Gallup, J., Karp-Lewis, S., et al. (2019). From the talking cure to a disease of silence. Effects of ethical violations in a psychoanalytic institute. *The International Journal of Psychoanalysis, 100*(2), 247–271.

Busch, B., Dill, H., & Mosser, P. (2020). Betroffene und ihr gesellschaftspolitisches Engagement gegen sexualisierte Gewalt. *Verhaltenstherapie & Psychosoziale Praxis, 52*(2), 317–327.

Caspari, C. (2012). *Shared decision making – Zwischen Wunsch und Wirklichkeit*. AV Akademikerverlag.

Caspari, P. (2021a). Aufdeckung als Prozess. In C. Fobian & R. Ulfers (Hrsg.), *Jungen als Betroffene sexualisierter Gewalt (Sexuelle Gewalt und Pädagogik)* (Bd. 7, 1. Aufl., S. 87–102.). Springer Fachmedien Wiesbaden GmbH; Springer VS.

Caspari, P. (2021b). *Gewaltpräventive Einrichtungskulturen. Theorie, Empirie, Praxis*. Springer VS.

Caspari, P., Dill, H., Hackenschmied, G., & Straus, F. (2021). *Ausgeliefert und verdrängt – Heimkindheiten zwischen 1949 und 1975 und die Auswirkungen auf die Lebensführung Betroffener. Eine begleitende Studie zur Bayerischen Anlauf- und Beratungsstelle für ehemalige Heimkinder* (Sexuelle Gewalt in Kindheit und Jugend: Forschung als Beitrag zur Aufarbeitung, 1. Aufl. 2021). Springer Fachmedien Wiesbaden.

Celenza, A. (1991). The misuse of countertransference love in sexual intimacies between therapists and patients. *Psychoanalytic Psychology, 8*(4), 501–509.

Christmann, B., & Wazlawik, M. (2019). Organisationsethik als Perspektive und Ausgestaltung von Schutzkonzepten gegen sexualisierte Gewalt in pädagogischen Einrichtungen. *Neue Praxis, 49*(3), 234–247.

Dausien, B. (1995). *Biographie und Geschlecht*. Dissertation.

Dehmers, J. (2011). *Wie laut soll ich denn noch schreien? Die Odenwaldschule und der sexuelle Missbrauch*. Rowohlt.

Devereux, G. (1984). *Angst und Methode in den Verhaltenswissenschaften*. Suhrkamp.

Diepold, B. (1994). Von der Psychagogik zur analytischen Kinderpsychotherapie. Vortrag zum 40 jährigen Bestehen des Göttinger Psychoanalytischen Instituts in Tiefenbrunn am 26.11.1994. http://www.diepold.de/barbara/von_der_psychagogik.pdf. Accessed: 11. März 2021.

Draucker, C. B., & Martsolf, D. S. (2008). Storying childhood sexual abuse. *Qualitative Health Research, 18*(8), 1034–1048.

Dreßing, H., Salize, H. J., Dölling, D., Hermann, D., Kruse, A., Schmitt, E., et al. (2018). Sexueller Missbrauch an Minderjährigen durch katholische Priester, Diakone und männliche Ordensangehörige im Bereich der Deutschen Bischofskonferenz, Projektbericht,

Mannheim, Heidelberg, Gießen. https://www.dbk.de/fileadmin/redaktion/diverse_downloads/dossiers_2018/MHG-Studie-gesamt.pdf. Accessed: 2. Apr. 2020.

Dührssen, A. (1962). Katamnestische Ergebnisse bei 1004 Patienten nach analytischer Psychotherapie. *Zeitschrift für psychosomatische Medizin, 8*, 94–113.

Dührssen, A. (1994). *Ein Jahrhundert psychoanalytische Bewegung in Deutschland: Die Psychotherapie unter dem Einfluß Freuds*. Vandenhoeck & Ruprecht.

Dührssen, A., & Jorswieck, E. (1965). Eine empirisch-statistische Untersuchung zur Leistungsfähigkeit psychoanalytischer Behandlung. *Der Nervenarzt, 36*, 166–169.

Enders, U. (2002). Institutionen und sexueller Missbrauch: Täterstrategien und Reaktionsweisen. In D. Bange & W. Körner (Hrsg.), *Handwörterbuch Sexueller Missbrauch* (S. 202–209). Hogrefe.

Enders, U. (2004). Traumatisierte Institutionen. Wenn eine Einrichtung zum Tatort sexueller Ausbeutung durch einen Mitarbeiter/eine Mitarbeiterin wurde. http://www.zartbitter.de/0/Eltern_und_Fachleute/6030_traumatisierte_institutionen.pdf. Accessed: 11. März 2021.

Enders, U., Kossatz, Y., Kelkel, M. & Eberhardt, B. (2010). Zur Differenzierung zwischen Grenzverletzungen, Übergriffen und strafrechtlich relevanten Formen der Gewalt im pädagogischen Alltag. Zugriff am 30.03.2020. http://www.praevention-bildung.dbk.de/fileadmin/redaktion/praevention/microsite/Downloads/Zartbitter_Grenzuebergriff-eStraftaten.pdf. Accessed: 30. März 2020.

Fahrig, H., Kronmüller, K. T., Hartmann, M., & Rudolf, G. (1996). Therapieerfolg analytischer Psychotherapie bei Kindern und Jugendlichen: Die Heidelberger Studie zur Analytischen Kinder- und Jugendlichen-Psychotherapie. *Zeitschrift für psychosomatische Medizin und Psychoanalyse, 42*(4), 375–395.

Fegert, J. M. (2006). Sexueller Missbrauch von Schutzbefohlenen und Abhängigen in Krankenbehandlung, Therapie und Pädagogik. In J. M. Fegert & M. Wolff (Hrsg.), *Sexueller Missbrauch durch Professionelle in Institutionen. Prävention und Intervention – ein Werkbuch* (2. Aktualisierte Aufl., S. 22–52).Juventa.

Fischer, G., & Riedesser, P. (2009). *Lehrbuch der Psychotraumatologie* (UTB Medizin, Psychologie, Bd. 8165, 4., aktualisierte und erweiterte Aufl.). Ernst Reinhardt Verlag. http://www.utb-studi-e-book.de/9783838581651

Flick, S. (2013). Paradoxien der Psychotherapie. Psychotherapeut_innen und die Kultur des Therapeutischen. *Freie Assoziation, 16*(3 und 4), 111–128.

Freud, S. (1912). *Ratschläge für den Arzt bei der psychoanalytischen Behandlung*. https://www.textlog.de/freud-psychoanalyse-ratschlaege-arzt-psychoanalytischen-behandlung.html. Accessed: 26. Febr. 2021.

Freud, S. (1914). *Bemerkungen über die Übertragungsliebe*. http://www.irwish.de/PDF/Psychologie/Freud/Freud-Bemerkungen_ueber_die_Uebertragungsliebe.pdf. Accessed: 27. Febr. 2021.

Freud, S. (1949 [1914]). *Bemerkungen über die Übertragungsliebe. (Weitere Ratschläge zur Technik der Psychoanalyse). Gesammelte Werke, Chronologisch geordnet* (Bd. 10. Werke aus den Jahren 1913–1917, S. 306–321) Imago Publishing Co Ltd. https://freud-online.de/index.php?page=445644700&f=1&i=445644700. Accessed: 15. Jan. 2021.

Gabbard, G. O. (1994). Sexual excitement and countertransference love in the analyst. *Journal of the American Psychoanalytic Association, 42*(4), 1083–1106.

Gartrell, N., Herman, J., Olarte, S., Feldstein, M., & Localio, R. (1987). Reporting practices of psychiatrists who knew of sexual misconduct by colleagues. *The American Journal of Orthopsychiatry, 57*(2), 287–295.

Geissler, B. (2013). *Professionalisierung und Profession. Zum Wandel klientenbezogener Berufe im Übergang zur post-industriellen Gesellschaft*. Die Hochschule, 1/2013. https://www.hoH.M.uni-halle.de/journal/texte/13_1/Geissler.pdf. Accessed: 11. März 2021.

Glaser, B. G. (1978). *Theoretical sensitivity (Advances in the Methodology of Grounded Theory)* Mill Valley Socioloty Press.

Glaser, B. G., & Strauss, A. L. (1967). *The discovery of grounded theory. Strategies for qualitative research*. Aldine.

Glaser, B. G., & Strauss, A. L. (1998). *Grounded theory*. Huber.

Glaser, B. G., & Strauss, A. L. (2009). *The discovery of grounded theory. Strategies for qualitative research* (4. paperback printing). Aldine.

Goffman, E. (1973). *Asyle. Über die soziale Situation psychiatrischer Patienten und anderer Insassen* (Edition Suhrkamp, Bd. 678). Suhrkamp.

Harvey, J. H., Orbuch, T. L., Chwalisz, K. D., & Garwood, G. (1991). Coping with sexual assault: The roles of account-making and confiding. *Journal of Traumatic Stress, 4*(4), 515–531.

Helfferich, C., Doll, D., Feldmann, J., & Kavemann, B. (2021). Sexuelle Übergriffe unter Jugendlichen als Frage von Macht, Geschlecht und sozialer Einbindung in Gruppen – eine qualitative Rekonstruktion. *Zeitschrift für Soziologie der Erziehung und Sozialisation, 41*(1), 73–89. https://content-select.com/de/portal/media/view/6012d05c-e63c-4b08-8b9e-7d18b0dd2d03. Accessed: 27. Febr. 2021.

Helming, E., Kindler, H., Langmeyer, A., Mayer, M., Entleitner, C., Mosser, P., et al. (Hrsg.). (2011). *Sexuelle Gewalt gegen Mädchen und Jungen in Institutionen*. München. http://www.dji.de/bibs/DJIAbschlussbericht_Sexuelle_Gewalt.pdf

Hermanns, H. (2003). Interviewen als Tätigkeit. In U. Flick, E. v. Kardorff, & I. Steinke (Hrsg.), *Qualitative Forschung. Ein Handbuch* (10. Aufl., S. 360–369). Rowohlt.

Heyne, C. (1991). *Tatort Couch. Sexueller Mißbrauch in der Therapie*. Kreuz.

Hirsch, M. (1997). Vernachlässigung, Misshandlung, Missbrauch im Rahmen einer psychoanalytischen Traumatologie. In U. T. Egle & A. v. Arnim (Hrsg.), *Sexueller Mißbrauch, Mißhandlung, Vernachlässigung. Erkennung und Behandlung psychischer und psychosomatischer Folgen früher Traumatisierungen; mit 22 Tabellen* (S. 103–116). Schattauer.

Hirsch, M. (2012). *„Goldmine und Minenfeld". Liebe und sexueller Machtmissbrauch in der analytischen Psychotherapie und anderen Abhängigkeitsbeziehungen* (Bibliothek der Psychoanalyse, Orig.-Ausg). Psychosozial-Verl.

Hirsch, M. (2018). *Das Phänomen Liebe. Wie sie entsteht, was sie in der Psychotherapie für Probleme macht und warum sie missbraucht werden kann*. Psychosozial-Verl.

Holroyd, J. C., & Brodsky, A. M. (1977). Psychologists' attitudes and practices regarding erotic and nonerotic physical contact with patients. *American Psychologist, 32*(10), 843–849.

Horn, H., Geiser-Elze, A., Reck, C., Hartmann, M., Stefini, A., Victor, D., et al. (2005). Zur Wirksamkeit psychodynamischer Kurzzeitpsychotherapie bei Kindern und Jugendlichen mit Depressionen. *Praxis der Kinderpsychologie und Kinderpsychiatrie, 54*(7), 578–597.

Hutterer-Krisch, R. (Hrsg.). (2007). *Grundriss der Psychotherapieethik. Praxisrelevanz, Behandlungsfehler und Wirksamkeit*. Springer. https://doi.org/10.1007/978-3-211-30671-0.

Institut für Psychotherapie und Psychoanalyse Heidelberg-Mannheim e. V. (1995). (Hrsg.), *Psychoanalyse im Widerspruch Heft13/95. Grenzüberschreitung. Missbrauch*. Selbstverlag.

Jaeggi, E., Faas, A., & Mruck, K. (2004). *Denkverbote gibt es nicht! Vorschlag zur interpretativen Auswertung kommunikativ gewonnener Daten. Forschungsbericht aus der Abteilung Psychologie im Institut für Sozialwissenschaften* (ISSN 1433-9218).

Jehle, J.-M. (2012). Attrition and Conviction Rates of Sexual Offences in Europe. Definitions and Criminal Justice Responses. *European Journal on Criminal Policy and Research, 18*(1), 145–161.

Kappler, S., Hornfeck, F., Pooch, M.-T., Kindler, H., & Tremel, I. (Deutsches Jugendinstitut, Hrsg.). (2019). *Kinder und Jugendliche besser schützen – Der Anfang ist gemacht. Schutzkonzepte gegen sexuelle Gewalt in den Bereichen: Bildung und Erziehung, Gesundheit, Freizeit. Abschlussbericht des Monitorings zum Stand der Prävention sexualisierter Gewalt an Kindern und Jugendlichen in Deutschland (2015–2018).* https://www.dji.de/fileadmin/user_upload/bibs2019/28116_UBSKM_DJI_Abschlussbericht.pdf. Accessed: 29. Sept. 2019.

Kaufman, K. L., & Erooga, M. (2016). *Risk profiles for institutional child sexual abuse. A literature review.* [Sydney, N.S.W.]: [Royal Commission into Institutional Responses to Child Sexual Abuse https://www.childabuseroyalcommission.gov.au/sites/default/files/file-list/Research%20Report%20-%20Risk%20profiles%20for%20institutional%20child%20sexual%20abuse%20-%20Causes.pdf?highcontrast=RegularContrast. Accessed: 9. Febr. 2019.

Kavemann, B., & Lohstöter, I. (1993). *Väter als Täter. Sexuelle Gewalt gegen Mädchen; „Erinnerungen sind wie eine Zeitbombe"* (rororo aktuell rororo Frauen, Bd. 5250, S. 56–60. Tsd). Rowohlt.

Kavemann, B., Graf-van Kesteren, A., Rothkegel, S., & Nagel, B. (Hrsg.). (2015a). *Erinnern, Schweigen und Sprechen nach sexueller Gewalt in der Kindheit Ergebnisse einer Interviewstudie mit Frauen und Männern, die als Kind sexuelle Gewalt erlebt haben.* Springer Fachmedien.

Kavemann, B., Rothkegel, S., & Nagel, B. (2015b). *Nicht aufklärbare Verdachtsfälle bei sexuellen Grenzverletzungen und sexualisierter Gewalt durch Mitarbeiter*innen in Institutionen.* Nicht 100 Prozent Sicherheit, aber 100 Prozent Professionalität. http://www.barbara-kavemann.de/download/2015_Broschuere_nicht_aufklaerbare_Verdachtsfaelle.pdf. Accessed: 11. Jan. 2019.

Kernberg, O. F., & Strauß, B. (Hrsg.). (2001). *Narzißtische Persönlichkeitsstörungen.* Mit 33 Tabellen (2., korr. Nachdr). Schattauer.

Keupp, H., Straus, F., Mosser, P., Gmür, W., & Hackenschmied, G. (2017a). *Schweigen – Aufdeckung – Aufarbeitung. Sexualisierte, psychische und physische Gewalt im Benediktinerstift Kremsmünster (Sexuelle Gewalt in Kindheit und Jugend).* Springer Fachmedien.

Keupp, H., Straus, F., Mosser, P., Gmür, W., & Hackenschmied, G. (2017b). *Sexueller Missbrauch und Misshandlungen in der Benediktinerabtei Ettal. Ein Beitrag zur wissenschaftlichen Aufarbeitung (Sexuelle Gewalt in Kindheit und Jugend).* Springer Fachmedien.

Keupp, H., Mosser, P., Hackenschmied, G., Busch, B., & Straus, F. (2019). *Die Odenwaldschule als Leuchtturm der Reformpädagogik und als Ort sexualisierter Gewalt. Eine sozialpsychologische Perspektive.* Springer Fachmedien.

Köhle, K., & Koerfer, A. (2011). Das Narrativ. In R. H. Adler, W. Herzog, P. Joraschky, K. Köhle, W. Langewitz, & T. v. Uexküll (Hrsg.), *Psychosomatische Medizin. Theo-*

retische Modelle und klinische Praxis (7., komplett überarb. Aufl., S. 359–375). Urban Fischer Verlag – Nachschlagewerke.

König, H.-D. (2003). Tiefenhermeneutik. In U. Flick, E. v. Kardorff, & I. Steinke (Hrsg.), *Qualitative Forschung. Ein Handbuch* (10. Aufl., S. 556–569). Rowohlt.

Körner, J. (1998a). Diskussion. *Forum der Psychoanalyse,14*, 341.

Körner, J. (1998b). Editorial. *Forum der Psychoanalyse,14*, 299–300.

Kreische, R. (1998). Psychoanalyse und staatliche Gesetze zur Verhinderung von sexuellem Missbrauch. *Forum der Psychoanalyse, 14*, 385–387.

Kronmüller, K.-T., Polstelnicu, I., Hartmann, M., Stefini, A., Geiser-Elze, A., Gerhold, M., et al. (2005). Zur Wirksamkeit psychodynamischer Kurzzeitpsychotherapie bei Kindern und Jugendlichen mit Angststörungen. *Praxis der Kinderpsychologie und Kinderpsychiatrie, 54*(7), 559–577.

Krutzenbichler, S. (1998). Lässt sich die psychoanalytische Ethik kodifizieren? *Forum der Psychoanalyse, 14*, 319–324.

Krutzenbichler, H. S., & Essers, H. (1991). *Muß denn Liebe Sünde sein? Über das Begehren des Analytikers*. Kore.

Kuckartz, U. (2012). *Qualitative Inhaltsanalyse. Methoden, Praxis, Computerunterstützung*. Beltz-Juventa.

Lockot, R. (2010). DPV und DPG auf dem dünnen Eis der DGPT. Zur Beziehungsgeschichte von Deutscher Psychoanalytischer Verinigung (DPV) und Deutscher Psychoanalytischer Gesellschaft (DPG) innerhalb der Deutschen Gesellschaft für Psychotherapie und Tiefenpsychologie (DGPT) bis 1967. *Psyche – Zeitschrift für Psychoanalyse und ihre Anwendungen, 64,* 1206–1242. https://dgpt.de/fileadmin/downloads/2-ueber_uns/geschichte-der-dgpt/Chronik_DPV_DPG_DGPT_Lockot.pdf. Accessed: 30. Jan. 2021.

Luhmann, N. (1994). *Soziale Systeme. Grundriß einer allgemeinen Theorie* (Suhrkamp-Taschenbuch Wissenschaft, Bd. 666, 5. Aufl.). Suhrkamp.

Maier-Kirstätter, C. (1995). Die „Lücke". In Institut für Psychotherapie und Psychoanalyse Heidelberg-Mannheim e. V. (Hrsg.), *Psychoanalyse im Widerspruch Heft13/95. Grenzüberschreitung* (S. 7–12). *Missbrauch*. Selbstverlag.

Maurer, S. (2018). Die Thematisierung sexualisierter Gewalt durch die „Neue Frauenbewegung". In A. Retkowski, A. Treibel, & E. Tuider (Hrsg.), *Handbuch sexualisierte Gewalt und pädagogische Kontexte* (S. 43–51). Beltz Juventa.

Mayring, P. (1983). *Qualitative Inhaltsanalyse. Grundlagen u. Techniken*. Beltz.

Mayring, P. (2015). *Qualitative Inhaltsanalyse. Grundlagen und Techniken* (Beltz Pädagogik, 12., überarb. Aufl.). Beltz. http://content-select.com/index.php?id=bib_view&ean=9783407293930

McNally, R. J. (2005). Debunking myths about trauma and memory. *Canadian Journal of Psychiatry, 50*(13), 817–822. http://journals.sagepub.com/doi/pdf/10.1177/070674370505001302. Accessed: 21. Jan. 2018

Merkens, H. (2003). Auswahlverfahren, Sampling, Fallkonstruktion. In U. Flick, E. v. Kardorff, & I. Steinke (Hrsg.), *Qualitative Forschung. Ein Handbuch* (10. Aufl., S. 286–299). Rowohlt.

Mitscherlich, A., & Mitscherlich, M. (2007). *Die Unfähigkeit zu trauern. Grundlagen kollektiven Verhaltens* (Piper, Bd. 168, 19. Aufl.). Piper.

Molitor, G. (1998). Diskussion. *Forum der Psychoanalyse,14*, 332.

Mosser, P. (2009). *Wege aus dem Dunkelfeld. Aufdeckung und Hilfesuche bei sexuellem Missbrauch an Jungen*. VS Verlag.

Mosser, P. (2012). *Sexuell grenzverletzende Kinder. Praxisansätze und ihre empirischen Grundlagen; eine Expertise für das IzKK – Informationszentrum Kindesmisshandlung/Kindesvernachlässigung (Wissenschaftliche Texte / Deutsches Jugendinstitut)*. DJI.

Mosser, P. (2018). Folgen und Nachwirkungen sexualisierter Gewalt. In A. Retkowski, A. Treibel, & E. Tuider (Hrsg.), *Handbuch sexualisierte Gewalt und pädagogische Kontexte* (im Erscheinen). Beltz Juventa.

Mosser, P. (2019). Auswirkungen sexualisierter Gewalt – Grundzüge einer sozialwissenschaftlichen Theorie unter einer bewältigungsorientierten Perspektive. In G. Stecklina & J. Wienforth (Hrsg.), *Soziale Arbeit und Lebensbewältigung. Grundlagen, Praxis, Kontroversen (Übergangs- und Bewältigungsforschung)*. Beltz Juventa.

Mosser, P. (2020). Handeln und Agieren als Formen der Ermächtigung – Betroffene von sexualisierter Gewalt auf ihrem Weg in die Öffentlichkeit. *Verhaltenstherapie & Psychosoziale Praxis, 52*(2), 331–350.

Mosser, P., & Hackenschmied, G. (2018). *Zeugnisse des Überlebens zur Aufarbeitung des Unrechts an Missbrauchsopfern in Heimen und Schulen. Soziale Arbeit – (K)Ein Ort für Menschenrechte?* Tutzing.

Mosser, P., & Schlingmann, T. (2013). Plastische Chirurgie an den Narben der Gewalt – Bemerkungen zur Medizinisierung des Traumabegriffs. *Forum Gemeindepsychologie, 18*(1).

Mosser, P., & Straus, F. (2020). Verlaufskurven der Bewältigung – Bedingungen des Umgangs mit Misshandlungs- und sexualisierten Gewalterfahrungen im institutionellen Kontext aus einer Lebenszeitperspektive. *Verhaltenstherapie & Psychosoziale Praxis, 52*(1), 103–109.

Mosser, P., Gmür, W., & Hackenschmied, G. (2018). Sozialwissenschaftliche Studien als Instrument zur Aufarbeitung sexualisierter Gewalt in Institutionen. In A. Retkowski, A. Treibel, & E. Tuider (Hrsg.), *Handbuch sexualisierte Gewalt und pädagogische Kontexte* (im Erscheinen). Beltz Juventa.

Oevermann, U. (1995). Die objektive Hermeneutik als unverzichtbare methologische Grundlage für die Analyse von Subjektivität. Zugleich eine Kritik der Tiefenhermeneutik. In T. Jung & S. Müller-Doohm (Hrsg.), *„Wirklichkeit" im Deutungsprozess. Verstehen und Methoden in den Kultur- und Sozialwissenschaften* (Suhrkamp-Taschenbuch Wissenschaft, Bd. 1048, 2. Aufl., S. 106–189). Suhrkamp.

Oppermann, C., Winter, V., Harder, C., Wolff, M., & Schröer, W. (Hrsg.). (2018). *Lehrbuch Schutzkonzepte in pädagogischen Organisationen. Mit Online-Materialien* (Studienmodule Soziale Arbeit, 1. Aufl). Beltz Juventa. http://www.content-select.com/index.php?id=bib_view&ean=9783779948360

Orbuch, T. L., Harvey, J. H., Davis, S. H., & Merbach, N. J. (1994). Account-making and confiding as acts of meaning in response to sexual assault. *Journal of Family Violence, 9*(3), 249–264.

Parin, P. (1978). Warum die Psychoanalytiker so ungern zu brennenden Zeitproblemen Stellung nehmen. Eine ethnologische Betrachtung. *Psyche, 32*(5/6), 385–399.

Pfadenhauer, M., & Sander, T. (2010). Professionssoziologie. In G. Kneer & M. Schroer (Hrsg.), *Handbuch spezieller Soziologien* (S. 361–378). Springer VS.

Pfannschmidt, H. (1998). Der „Gebrauch der Lüste“ in der Analysestunde. Oder: Warum es so schwer zu sein scheint, Psychoanalyse und Erotik unter einen Hut zu bekommen. *Forum der Psychoanalyse,14*, 364–384.

Pope, K. S., & Bouhoutsos, J. C. (1994). *Als hätte ich mit einem Gott geschlafen. Sexuelle Beziehungen zwischen Therapeuten und Patienten* (Goldmann, Bd. 12463, Ungekürzte Taschenbuchausg) Goldmann.

Reichertz, J. (2003). Objektive Hermeneutik und hermeneutische Wissensoziologie. In U. Flick, E. v. Kardorff, & I. Steinke (Hrsg.), *Qualitative Forschung. Ein Handbuch* (10. Aufl., S. 514–524). Rowohlt.

Retkowski, A., Treibel, A., & Tuider, E. (2018). Einleitung: Pädagogische Kontexte und Sexualisierte Gewalt. In A. Retkowski, A. Treibel, & E. Tuider (Hrsg.), *Handbuch sexualisierte Gewalt und pädagogische Kontexte* (S. 15–30). Beltz Juventa.

Rieske, T. V., Scambor, E., Wittenzellner, U., Könnecke, B., & Puchert, R. (Hrsg.). (2018). *Aufdeckungsprozesse männlicher Betroffener von sexualisierter Gewalt in Kindheit und Jugend. Verlaufsmuster und hilfreiche Bedingungen* (Sexuelle Gewalt und Pädagogik, Bd. 4). Springer Fachmedien Wiesbaden. https://doi.org/10.1007/978-3-658-15803-3.

Rohne, H.-C., & Wirths, A.-C. (2018). Die Entwicklung des Sexualstrafrechts in der Bundesrepublik Deutschland. In A. Retkowski, A. Treibel, & E. Tuider (Hrsg.), *Handbuch sexualisierte Gewalt und pädagogische Kontexte* (S. 90–100). Beltz Juventa.

Rosenthal, G. (1987). *… Wenn alles in Scherben fällt …“. Von Leben und Sinnwelt der Kriegsgeneration* (Biographie und Gesellschaft, Bd. 6). VS Verlag. https://doi.org/10.1007/978-3-663-09168-4.

Rosenthal, G., & Fischer-Rosenthal, W. (2003). Analyse narrativ-biographischer Interviews. In U. Flick, E. v. Kardorff, & I. Steinke (Hrsg.), *Qualitative Forschung. Ein Handbuch* (10. Aufl., S. 456–468). Rowohlt.

Rutter, P. (1990). *Sex in the forbidden zone. When men in power-therapists, doctors, clergy, teachers, and others-betray women's trust*. Unwin.

Sandler, A., & Godley, W. (2004). Institutional responses to boundary violations. The case of Masud Khan. *The International Journal of Psychoanalysis, 85*(1), 27–43.

Schleu, A. (2021). *Umgang mit Grenzverletzungen. Professionelle Standards und ethische Fragen in der Psychotherapie* (Psychotherapie: Praxis, 1. Aufl. 2021). Springer Berlin: Springer.

Schleu, A., & Habenicht, I. (Hrsg.). (2014). *Verwickeln und Entwickeln. Ethische Fragen in der Psychotherapie*. VAS.

Schleu, A., Tibone, G., Gutmann, T., & Thorwart, J. (2018). Sexueller Missbrauch in der Psychotherapie. Notwendige Diskussion der Perspektiven von Psychotherapeuten und Juristen. *Psychotherapeutenjournal, 17*(1), 11–19. https://www.psychotherapeutenjournal.de/ptk/web.nsf/gfx/88268FE43120BEABC125825E0041B949/$file/PTJ_1_2018_Artikel%20Schleu%20et%20al.pdf. Accessed: 25. Febr. 2021

Schuhrke, B. (2002). Sexuell auffälliges Verhalten von Kindern. In D. Bange & W. Körner (Hrsg.), *Handwörterbuch sexueller Missbrauch* (S. 542–547). Hogrefe Verl. für Psychologie.

Slochower, J. (2017). Introduction to panel. Ghosts that haunt—Sexual boundary violations in our communities. *Psychoanalytic Dialogues, 27*(1), 61–66.

Sonnenmoser, M. (2002). *Psychotherapieforschung: Stiefkind Prozessforschung* (PP!, Ausgabe April 2002, S. 153). Ärzteblatt. https://www.aerzteblatt.de/archiv/33456/Psychotherapieforschung-Stiefkind-Prozessforschung. Accessed: 11. Febr. 2021.

Spieß, H.-H. (1998). Diskussion. *Forum der Psychoanalyse,14*, 339.

Stichweh, R. (2005). *Die Soziologie der Professionen. Zur Zukunft einer Forschungstradition und einer Semantik der Selbstbeschreibung*. https://www.fiw.uni-bonn.de/demokratieforschung/personen/stichweh/papers. Accessed: 25. Febr. 2021.

therapie.de. (n.d.). *Wo kann man eine Beschwerde über seinen Therapeuten einlegen?* https://www.therapie.de/psyche/info/fragen/beschwerden-in-der-psychotherapie/moeglichkeiten-und-wege/. Accessed: 11. März 2021.

Tibone, G., & Schmieder-Dembek, B. (2015). Abstinenz und AbstinenzverletzunFunktion enthobengen in der psychoanalytischen Ausbildung. *Forum der Psychoanalyse, 31*(1), 17–34.

Tschan, W. (2005). *Missbrauchtes Vertrauen. Sexuelle Grenzverletzungen in professionellen BeziehungenUrsachen und Folgen* (2., neu bearbeitete und erweiterte Aufl.). S. Karger.

Twemlow, S. W., & Gabbard, G. O. (1989). The lovesick therapist. In G. O. Gabbard (Hrsg.), Sexual Exploitation in Professional Relationships (S. 71–87). Washington, DC: American Psychiatric Press.

Unabhängige Aufarbeitungskommission. (2017). *Geschichten, die zählen. Zwischenbericht*. https://www.aufarbeitungskommission.de/wp-content/uploads/2017/06/Zwischenbericht_Aufarbeitungskommission_Juni_2017.pdf. Accessed: 30. Sept. 2020.

Unabhängige Aufarbeitungskommission. (2019a). *Geschichten, die zählen. Bilanzbericht* (Bd. 1). https://www.aufarbeitungskommission.de/wp-content/uploads/2019/05/Bilanzbericht_2019_Band-I.pdf. Accessed: 6. Aug. 2020.

Unabhängige Aufarbeitungskommission. (2019b). *Rechte und Pflichten: Aufarbeitungsprozesse in Institutionen*. https://www.aufarbeitungskommission.de/wp-content/uploads/2020/04/Empfehlungen-Aufarbeitung-sexuellen-Kindesmissbauchs_Aufarbeitungskommission-2020.pdf. Accessed: 6. Aug. 2020.

VAKJP. (2001). *Ethik-Leitlinien der VAKJP. in der Fassung des Beschlusses der Mitgliederversammlung am 30.4.2001*. https://www.vakjp.de/pdf/ethikleitlinien.pdf. Accessed: 27. Febr. 2021.

Vogd, W. (2005). *Systemtheorie und rekonstruktive Sozialforschung. Eine empirische Versöhnung unterschiedlicher theoretischer Perspektiven*. Budrich. Verfügbar unter http://deposit.dnb.de/cgi-bin/dokserv?id=2662437&prov=M&dok_var=1&dok_ext=htm

Vogt, I. (1991). Konsequenzen für Therapie und Praxis. Forschungsergebnisse. In Arbeitsgemeinschaft „Frauen in der psychosozialen Versorgung“ der DGVT (Hrsg.), *Sexuelle Übergriff in der Therapie. Kunstfehler oder Kavaliersdelikt? Dokumentation des öffentlichen Hearings am 19. Januar 1991 in Bonn* (S. 63–70). DGVT.

Wallace, E. M. (2007). Losing a training analyst for ethical violations. A candidate's perspective. *The International Journal of Psychoanalysis, 88*(Pt 5), 1275–1288.

Weick, K. E., Sutcliffe, K. M., & Burkhardt, S. (2016). *Das Unerwartete managen. Wie Unternehmen aus Extremsituationen lernen* (3. Aufl.). Poeschl.

Welzer, H. (2002). *Das kommunikative Gedächtnis. Eine Theorie der Erinnerung*. Beck. http://hsozkult.geschichte.hu-berlin.de/rezensionen/2003-3-147

Welzer, H., Moller, S., & Tschuggnall, K. (2015). *„Opa war kein Nazi“. Nationalsozialismus und Holocaust im Familiengedächtnis* (Fischer Die Zeit des Nationalsozialismus, Bd. 15515, Originalausgabe, 9. Aufl.). Fischer-Taschenbuch.

Wenger, E. (2008). *Communities of practice. Learning, meaning, and identity (Learning in doing)*. Cambridge University Press.

Wilson, J. P., Drozdek, B., & Turkovic, S. (2006). Posttraumatic shame and guilt. *Trauma, Violence & Abuse, 7*(2), 122–141.

Winkelmann, K., Hartmann, M., Neumann, K., Hennch, C., Reck, C., Victor, D., et al. (2000). Stabilität des Therapieerfolgs nach analytischer Kinder-und Jugendlichen-Psychotherapie – Eine Fünf-Jahres-Katamnese. *Praxis der Kinderpsychologie und Kinderpsychiatrie, 49*(5), 315–328.

Wirtz, U. (1994). Therapie als sexuelles Agierfeld. In K. M. Bachmann & W. Bröker (Hrsg.), *Sexueller Mißbrauch in Psychotherapie und Psychiatrie* (S. 33–44). Huber.

Wittgenstein, L., & Kenny, A. (Hrsg.). (1996). *Ein Reader* (Universal-Bibliothek, Bd. 9470, 1. Aufl.). Reclam.

Wolff, S. (2003). Dokumenten- und Aktenanalyse. In U. Flick, E. v. Kardorff, & I. Steinke (Hrsg.), *Qualitative Forschung. Ein Handbuch* (10. Aufl., S. 502–514). Rowohlt.

Wruck, P. (1998). Diskussion. Forum der Psychoanalyse,14, 339–340.

The manufacturer's authorised representative in the EU is Springer Nature Customer Service Centre GmbH, Europaplatz 3, 69115 Heidelberg, Germany. If you have any concerns regarding our products, please contact ProductSafety@springernature.com

Printed and bound by CPI Group (UK) Ltd, Croydon, CR0 4YY
28/09/2026
02224076-0001